3000 800026 14
St. Louis Community College

D1624656

FPCC
APR 19 1993

 St. Louis Community
College

Forest Park
Florissant Valley
Meramec

Instructional Resources
St. Louis, Missouri

INVENTORY 98

LIFE, DEATH, AND IN BETWEEN

Also by Harold L. Klawans

Trials of An Expert Witness
Newton's Madness
Toscanini's Fumble
The Medicine of History
Sins of Commission
Informed Consent
The Jerusalem Code
Deadly Medicine (U.K.)

LIFE, DEATH, AND IN BETWEEN

TALES OF CLINICAL NEUROLOGY

Harold L. Klawans, MD

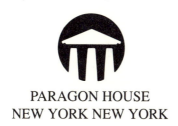

PARAGON HOUSE
NEW YORK NEW YORK

First edition, 1992

Published in the United States by

Paragon House Publishers
90 Fifth Avenue
New York, NY 10011

Copyright © 1992 by Harold L. Klawans

All rights reserved. No part of this book may be reproduced, in any
form, without written permission from the publishers, unless by a
reviewer who wishes to quote brief passages.

Although all the case studies featured in this book are true, in many
instances the names and identifying characteristics of contemporary subjects have been changed to protect the privacy of those
individuals.

"Case History" is used by permission of its author and is from the
book *White Coat, Purple Coat,* published by Persea Books, New York,
1991.

Library of Congress Cataloging-in-Publication Data
Klawans, Harold L.
Life, death, and in between : tales of clinical neurology / Harold L. Klawans.
1st ed.
        p. cm.
ISBN 1-55778-526-0
1. Neurology—Popular works. 2. Neurology—Case studies.
I. Title
RC346.K53   1992
616.8—dc20   92-4663
                                                   CIP

ISBN 1-55778-526-0

Manufactured in the United States of America

To Barbara
With my love

and to Andy and Emily
and Debby, Becky and Brad, and Jonathan
With our love

CONTENTS

For the patient will live
and you will try to understand

or the patient will not live
and you will try to understand

John Stone, MD
Gaudeamus Igitur: A Valediction

PREFACE

Looking back, I realize that becoming a real doctor was the most difficult achievement of my life. I hope other physicians make that transition far more quickly than I did, far more easily. I'm a neurologist. And neurologists, for generations, were not real doctors. We were consultants, consulting neurologists. We didn't actually take care of sick people. Others did that. These tales are about patients I met along the way and whose stories, personalities, fates, reactions, helped make me into a real doctor, one who no longer takes a history, performs an examination, makes a diagnosis, suggests a course of management, and then closes the door. My role as a real doctor, I've only learned over the years.

That role has nothing to do with the problems of American medicine. Not the *big problems,* not the so-called crises, not the ones that make all the headlines. What concerns me are those issues that directly affect what happens between the patient and me. That is what medicine should be all about, that series of one-on-one individual interactions. Human interactions that may or may not have medical significance but often have human significance. And that human significance is not just for the patient. Far from it.

That is what this book is about. Those individual situations, individual patients, individual crises that have altered or affected how I think and feel about medicine, and about myself and the way I interact with patients. Thirty years ago I chose neurology as a career not only because I was fascinated by the brain but also as a defense against what I did not yet know how to do—take care of sick people. Today I spend most of my life giving chronic care to patients with severe debilitating neurological diseases, trying to help them and their families cope with all the problems and complications of these disorders.

Medicine has changed over these three decades, but the problems remain the problems of illness, dependency, facing death, coming to terms with disability and mortality. These are not strictly medical problems. They are ethical, moral, social, and above all human problems. The true practice of medicine has always been difficult. It's not that it's more difficult today, but it is different. Patients' needs are not different, but their expectations are and so are their frustrations. And so too are the expectations and frustrations of the physicians. All too often, physicians escape the demands of their patients by withdrawing into the business aspects of medicine, and patients similarly withdraw. Such withdrawal creates separate camps that seem to be at odds with each other.

I'm not the same person I was when I haltingly put my stethoscope to the chest of a real, live patient for the first time. I certainly am not the same physician I was when I examined my first admission as an intern, not when the first patient with Parkinson's disease came into my office. The process of being a physician has changed me and will undoubtedly continue to change me. Some of those changes revolve around certain individual patients whose stories are the stuff of this book.

The collection opens with the various stages of my training. Once that training was over, my career as a treating physician really began. That is what has occupied me for most of the last twenty-four years and, appropriately, that is what occupies most of the book. The organization follows whatever logic there has been in the organization of my professional life, trying to group together those experiences that had to do with research and those that had to do with other aspects of taking care of sick people.

"Tell me, Dr. Klawans," the lawyer began his cross-examination. "How do you spend your day? Do you have a private practice? Don't you just teach and do research?"

It was a line of questioning I'd expected. I was an expert witness. One way to attack me and my opinion was to show the jury that I was not really a doctor.

I tried to explain my life. I had a private practice. I saw my own patients. Some I'd been seeing for more than twenty years. Yes, sometimes I saw them with medical students, but I always saw and talked to my patients on each and every office visit. And yes, I did research on them. On my own patients.

"So they are merely guinea pigs?" he persisted.

"I wish they were," I said.

"And why is that?"

"Then it wouldn't hurt if they didn't get better."

Clinical research, like the good old days, just isn't what it used to be. When I first started out, the approval process was such a simple one. Half the time I just talked my idea over with the chairman as we drank a cup of espresso in his office. Now a defined process and bureaucracy have been put in place to ensure that the rights of the patient are protected, so that it now can take months to get a protocol approved. Are the patients' rights protected any better?

The patient is sick. The patient is desperate. I have this new drug, this new surgical procedure. Will it be the miracle he seeks? That is the only important question. And it is never asked. The process itself supplies the answer.

My first research patient, the first one to take levodopa, asked two questions.

"Will I get better?"

I told him that I hoped he would, but explained that I could promise nothing. That was all I said, but it was not what he heard nor what he felt. I was his doctor. Would I be doing this if it wasn't going to help him? And help him a lot?

He knew his miracle was just around the corner.

"Is it safe?"

I explained the risks.

"I knew it'd be safe. You wouldn't give it to me if it wasn't, would you?"

I gave him a simple sheet to sign and so we got started together.

Today, I hand out a brochure put together by our research team, the drug company, the hospital's lawyers and ethicists, and approved by the Committee on Human Investigation. I ask the patient to read it, study it.

The patient glances at it and asks two questions: "Will I get better, Doc? Is it safe?" The same two questions.

I give the same two answers. Institutionalization offers no assurance of protection of patient rights. What is required are physicians who protect the rights of desperate patients, who place patients first. Not science, not progress, not career advancement, but the patient. That is not always easy. Do not desperate situations demand desperate solutions?

Are not desperate patients willing to go anywhere? To try anything?

Many are.

So they have to be protected. And their doctor cannot, by himself, decide what is good for them. For he, too, may be desperate.

So who can make the decision? Who can protect the patient from himself? From his doctor?

A committee.

It's the American Way.

Does it work? Perhaps.

Is there a better way?

Of course. The patient should never need to be protected from his own doctor. The doctor must protect his patient at all times. If only that could always be true.

For more than a decade I have pursued two professions, medicine and literature. It has been a joint pursuit not without its cost. I thought I could add the second without endangering the first. I was wrong. I've been misled. Chekhov has lied to me. His oft-quoted observation is an absurdity, an out-and-out lie:

> You advised me not to pursue two hares at a time and to abandon the practice of medicine . . . . I feel more contented and more satisfied when I realize that I have two professions, not one. Medicine is my lawful wife and literature my mistress. When I grow weary of one, I pass the night with the other. This may seem disorderly, but it is not dull, and besides, neither of them suffers because of my infidelity. If I did not have my medical work, it would be hard to give my thought and liberty of spirit to literature.

What an outlandish statement. No reader could take this seriously and certainly no writer and certainly no man's wife. Writing, good writing, requires intense, almost libidinal effort. If you put that energy into writing something else will have to suffer from not receiving that effort, that intensity, that portion of your libidinal energy. The fact is that Chekhov was not married at the time he tried juggling his two careers. He only got married years after he'd given up practicing medicine to devote all of his time and energy to the pursuit of writing.

Has my professional life as a physician suffered? Yes. I could be like Chekhov and point out that I see more patients now than I ever did, or . . . . But why lie? At one time I sustained an academic career

4

that included teaching, patient care, clinical research, and basic science research. I ran a laboratory that was on the cutting edge. I still teach. I still do clinical research. You've already heard about my patients. I haven't been inside "my" lab in a decade. So much for the cutting edge.

But writing has also enriched my life. And, I hope, the lives of my patients. It has made me even more aware of all the stories around me, the narrative of each patient's life. Not just the narrative of his disease. I had always wanted to know each patient's history, the history of his or her disease, a history of sickness, a tale of illness, that unique narrative of clues and suffering. But now I need to know much more, for the true history lead both to sickness and to coping with that sickness, to weaknesses and to strength, to perceptions and adaptations, to the unique humanity that houses a unique form of illness.

In a recent issue of *Modern Painters,* I came across a review of a new book entitled *The Art of Death: Visual Culture in the English Death Ritual*, by Nigel Llewellyn. Marc Jordan, a deputy editor of *The Dictionary of Art*, wrote that "death . . . has gone into the twilight world of the hospital ward and the nursing home. Few people now die surrounded by the familiar objects and faces among which they lived."

Jordan was right. Far too few people are allowed to die at home, especially in America, and that is both tragic and perverse. It contributes to many of our social and medical problems, including the inordinate cost of medical care in this country. A hugely disproportionate amount of the overall cost of medical care is assessed in the last month of life, all too often only to transform that month of life into thirty days of prolonged death.

Yet does *Neurology* lament this issue? Does *The New England Journal of Medicine*? I am far more likely to read about it in *Modern Painters*. The isolation of death. The removal of dying from the living, from the life of that dying person. The depersonalization and institutionalization of dying. This distinction does little good to anyone and much harm individually and institutionally. We, as individuals and as a society, no longer are allowed to experience death as the natural conclusion of life, not even when we ourselves enter into that last good night. And when we enter it, we go alone, isolated from every vestige of whatever it was that gave meaning to our lives.

So, of course we struggle. It cannot end like this. Life had to mean more than that. Our doctors must struggle. They must fight. Modern medicine must put up a battle. A raging battle: Rage! Rage!

"We did everything we could," the doctor says. Then the litany. CPR. Ventilators. Defibrillation. For three days. But. . . the voice trails off.

Yet the patient was eighty-seven. She hadn't wanted to come to the hospital in the first place. She had cancer. She knew she could never be cured, that she would only get worse. She knew. Her doctor knew. Her family knew. She had been ready to die. She had come to terms with that fact.

"We did everything . . . ."

He had done nothing, but nothing is not something Medicine and its practitioners do very well.

Why not?

It is as if we have created a new mystery religion. A new ritual that we can graft onto any form of religion without being accused of heresy. A mystery with its own truth that can only be learned through a ritual of revelation and that revelation can only occur within the sanctuaries of one of its own cathedrals, with at least one of the high priests in attendance, white-coated, of course.

Like all religious rituals, it produces awe. And wonder. And faith. And doubts. Faith and frustration. Anger, anger at the God or gods.

How could they let this happen?

How could they let her die?

How could they take her away? They did that. They gave up. They set the rules, played the game, and blew the final whistle. They are the timekeepers. Yet doctors do not cause death. The pronouncement of death is not what ends life.

Dead is dead. No ventilator can change that.

These stories all took place. The names have all been changed. So have many of the details of the patients' lives, but not the science nor the medicine, and not the essence of what happened to the patients and their doctor.

LIFE, DEATH, AND IN BETWEEN

PART ONE

COMING OF AGE IN AMERICA

The very first day of medical school we go into an anatomy lab and stick a knife into that cadaver. That's not a normal human act. And once we do that we're different. We develop a shell around ourselves.

Edward Rosenbaum, MD

1

THE MAN WITHOUT A HISTORY

History is a guide to navigation in perilous times.

David C. McCullough

My internship started at 4:00 P.M. on the last Thursday of June 1962. The rest of the interns and I had arrived at the hospital by noon. We were fed lunch, given our uniforms (white slacks, short white jackets, and short white smocks of the type now relegated solely to pharmacists and dental students), led on a short tour through the hospital, forced to sit through any number of introductory speeches (none short enough to be tolerable or with sufficient information to be worthwhile), and then taken to our initial posts or rotations. Twelve of us were medical interns. That meant that we would spend all twelve months of that year working on medical services with medical patients. No surgery. No obstetrics or gynecology. No pediatrics. That was the first year that there had ever been such medical internships in Illinois. Prior to that year, all interns took what were called rotating internships, a year spent oscillating back and forth from one service to another with two- to four-week stops on everything from anesthesiology to X-ray.

Most interns still did that, but not us. We would have six two-month assignments. Four on medical wards, one in the Intensive Care Unit, and one in psychiatry. Two of us would be on each rotation together and we'd split night call. That meant that one of the pair would be in the hospital every night. That translated into a schedule of thirty-six hours on duty followed by twelve hours off duty. Thirty-six on/twelve off, every other night for 365 days. Either 187 or 188 nights in the hospital, trying to get a few hours of sleep in the on-call rooms. Then the twelve medical interns would go on to residencies in Internal Medicine. At least that's what the other eleven would do. I would go on to do a residency in Neurology. Everyone already knew that. I was not a pariah, but I was not one of them. I was an outsider, a stranger in a strange land.

At 4:00 P.M. I went to my assigned ward, an acute medical ward. I met my fellow medical intern and my medical resident, and the three of us made walking rounds. There were forty-seven beds and forty-six patients. There could only be one admission that night. But which of us would be on call?

I was the logical one, the resident said. I was from Chicago. I had spent many months at the hospital as a medical student and already knew my way around the place. I should take call the first night. Besides, the other resident was exhausted; he had driven all the way from Pittsburgh by himself.

So I took the call. I realized full well that that meant I'd do 188 nights during the next year, not 187, but I'd still survive. Probably.

The other intern went home. The resident and I spent another two hours reviewing the twenty-three patients for whom I would have primary intern responsibility. The diversity of diseases and problems were enough to make my head spin: diabetes, recovering heart attacks, hepatitis, bleeding ulcers, strokes. That should not have surprised me. I'd chosen to take my medical residency here for that very reason. It was a hospital made up of general medical wards, not a series of subspecialty services. General medical wards are just that —wards filled with patients who were a mixture of every possible type of disease. Other hospitals had specialty wards and the interns went from one service to another. Three weeks on diabetes, two on the liver service, four for cardiology. That wasn't for me. I was going to go directly from one year of learning general medicine to a lifetime in Neurology. I didn't want a taste of medical subspecialization. I needed as much general medicine as I could get. I wanted to spend my first year inundated by every medical disease there was. It was not the specialist approach I needed, but something far more basic. I needed to learn how to take care of sick people, how to make critical decisions. How to recognize that critical decisions had to be made. How to be comfortable with disease, with sick patients.

How to be a doctor.

That I had not learned in medical school. In medical school, I learned facts about disease: Biochemical facts. Anatomical facts. Pathological facts. Physiological facts. Facts that were only a starting place, since most of them would change in the next two decades.

12

Facts and a method. A method to examine patients. To take a history from patients and examine them. To begin to learn how to observe. To make observations as to health and disease, observations that are still valid today.

But I learned nothing about patients. I cannot today recall a single patient I saw in medical school.

And even less about making decisions, about taking responsibility. It wasn't mine to take then. But now it was.

I was an intern. And soon I'd have my first patient.

How soon?

It was almost 9:00 P.M.

And what would this patient have?

He couldn't be too sick. After all, it was a scheduled admission, not an acute emergency.

"Let's find out about your patient," my resident said, as if he had been reading my mind.

"We can do that?"

He nodded and led me down to medical admissions and there on a clipboard was a list of medical admissions for that night. My patient was the first one on the list.

His name was Hartung. William Hartung.

His age was listed as sixty-two.

His diagnosis was coma.

That was not a routine admission. That was a medical emergency. Why was he in coma?

"That's your job," my resident said, once again reading my mind. "He won't be here until one o'clock. I'm going home. If you need help, call me. But you shouldn't. This is right up your alley."

"My alley?"

"Sure. Coma is a neurologic problem. The brain isn't able to maintain consciousness. It's neurology. All you have to do is figure out why the brain isn't working."

Call if you need help?

If? What did I know about coma? I was just an intern, not a neurologist. And I'd only been an intern for five hours.

Some possible causes bounced into my head. Even my short list was long, everything from a stroke to liver failure. And I was certain the real list, the list that any experienced doctor could conjure up on demand was far longer. I had to know what my patient might have. If William Hartung went into coma because of some disease I hadn't thought about, the odds were I wouldn't be able to make that

13

diagnosis. And without a diagnosis, we wouldn't be able to help him. And it'd be my fault.

I needed to know the differential diagnoses of coma, the complete differential diagnoses. That list of all the possible causes and how to tell one from the other. How? Where?

That I knew. French's *Differential Diagnosis*. It was a textbook of such listings with comprehensive discussions. I had three hours or more. I could go to the library, which was open to midnight.

It took me less than three minutes to walk to the library and less than that once there to locate the book and plant myself in a study carrel and set to work. The differential diagnoses of coma, with forty pages with six tables but no illustrations.

I read the forty pages through once and then went back, putting together my own working list of what I had to do. The first part of the list was history. The questions I had to ask about his past medical history, facts I needed to know because those facts influenced the possibilities of various diagnoses.

Had he ever been in a hospital before?

If so, for what?

Did he have high blood pressure?

Heart disease?

Liver disease?

Was he on any medication?

Which ones?

Had he stopped taking them?

It took me an hour to finish my list. I knew just what I had to ask. But of whom? Not William Hartung. He was in coma.

His wife. She'd have to be coming with him. She wouldn't let her husband come to a hospital alone. No wife would. Not a husband who was in coma at one o'clock in the morning. I'd ask his wife. If he was married. And she was alive. With my luck, he'd be a widower.

I'd ask his kids.

Or worse, a bachelor.

His girlfriend. Or boyfriend.

A recluse. He could be a recluse. With no friends at all.

But I needed a history. I could feel the panic heightening. Someone will be with him. But what if he comes alone? How can I find out anything?

How? His medical records.

He was coming to our hospital. We had to be his hospital. His doctor admitted his patients there. Maybe this wasn't his first admission. All I needed was his old records. Then I'd know his entire history. I'd be waiting at the gate, armed with facts.

I called medical records.

As soon as a patient was put on the admission list, all of his old records were sent to the floor where he was to be admitted.

"Hartung," I asked. "William Hartung. Did you send his records to Eleven East?"

"No."

"No? Why not?"

There weren't any. This was his first admission.

No records.

No past history.

No facts.

I would not be armed. I'd be naked. I could feel the sweat streaming down from my armpits. There had to be some way to get some facts, to feel less naked.

Something.

Anything.

There was.

His doctor. I'd call his doctor. The doctor had to know why he was admitting his patient. He had to know the past medical history. His doctor. I'd call his doctor.

Relief.

My heart rate slowed. I went back to the Medical Admitting Office and looked at the list. William Hartung was still number one on the list. He was still sixty-two years old and according to the list he was still in coma and still would be when he got here from some small town in Wisconsin at 1:00 A.M. And his doctor was Joe Staley. I knew him. I'd worked up several of his patients when I was a junior medical student. He was a nice guy. He wouldn't mind if I called, even if it was a quarter to twelve. What a relief.

I called and told him who I was and that I'd be taking care of William Hartung.

"What's he got?" Dr. Staley asked me.

"I don't know. He's not here yet."

"Then why are you calling me?"

I explained.

He couldn't help me. He didn't know the patient. The patient's brother was his next-door neighbor. Dr. Staley knew nothing at all about William Hartung's history except that he'd never been to see a doctor.

"A healthy guy."

"I don't know that."

"But he's never ever seen a physician."

"That's because he's a Christian Scientist."

A Christian Scientist! So much for an accurate medical history from his doctor.

I was no longer sweating. I was beyond sweating. I looked at the clock. Eleven fifty-five. The library would close in five minutes and I hadn't finished my notes about the physical exam in coma.

My notes!

They were still in the library. I slammed the phone back down and raced back to the library.

It was still open. The book was still there, right where I'd left it. So were my notes. Unfinished. I had only an hour to go. I went back to work on what to do in examining a patient in coma. Not just any patient. My patient. William Hartung. The man without a history.

The lights went out.

A power failure! That was all I needed.

And back on.

Thank God for the reserve generator.

And off again.

And on again.

The library was closing. It was midnight, but I had to finish my notes. I had to be ready for William Hartung.

He would be on Eleven East in an hour. And I had to be there to take care of him. Ready or not. I had to be ready. I took French's and headed out the door.

"Doctor."

The voice froze me in my steps. It was the librarian. The Wicked Witch of the West who protected the library. She never lost a book. Never, and she was not about to start.

She weighed less than a hundred pounds. Half what I weighed. I could hit her over the head with French's and then leave. They'd never know who did it. They'd never convict me. I needed that book.

"Doctor."

Or bolt.

Run.

She was ninety years old. She'd never be able to catch me.

"Doctor Klawans."

She knew my name. How?

Maybe she really was a witch with strange supernatural powers.

16

"Give me that book."

I turned. Defeated. I handed it to her. Speechless.

She took the book.

I needed it.

Without it, I was lost.

She opened it, took out the card, wrote something on it, my name I suppose, and handed the book back to me.

"Forty-eight hours," she smiled.

"Thank you," I blurted.

"Good luck," she said.

"How?" I asked.

"They send me pictures of all the interns."

I stood there. Fixed in place.

She turned off the lights. The library was closed. It was midnight.

One hour to go.

I raced to the elevator and got up to Eleven East. The nurse was at the nursing station. Had Mr. Hartung been admitted yet? My Mr. Hartung?

No.

Was he still scheduled?

Yes.

When?

One. I had less than an hour left. Back to French's.

More reading.

More notes.

More lists.

I had to be ready, to be prepared.

At twelve-fifty-five the nurse tapped me on the shoulder. I wasn't ready yet. He wasn't supposed to arrive until one o'clock. I had five more minutes.

He had arrived.

Godot, without a history.

Five more minutes. I thought to myself.

"He's in Eleven twenty-three."

Just five more minutes.

"And he is in coma."

"Oh, my God."

"His wife is with him."

God was not all bad. I could get some history, some facts. I sat there staring at my notes.

"Doctor," she said. She was in her forties. She'd been a nurse at this hospital for twenty years. She'd been through this before with twenty classes of new interns.

"Doctor," she repeated.

I got up and picked up my black bag. "Eleven twenty-three," I said.

She nodded.

I knew just what to do. I'd examine him from top to bottom. I'd start by palpating his skull, to make certain that there was no evidence of head trauma, that no one had hit him on the head with a sledgehammer. Next came the eyes. The sclera. Were they yellow because of jaundice? Or pale because of anemia? The pupils. Size, shape. How they reacted to light. My list was almost endless. It concluded with his toes. Were they club-shaped because of chronic lung disease?

"His wife," the nurse said.

"What?"

"His wife. She wants to talk to you."

A wife that could talk. There would be some history.

When I got to 1123, William Hartung was lying in the bed, breathing quietly. I counted the rate. Eighteen breaths per minute. No respiratory disease. No need for a ventilator.

I introduced myself to the wife, noting a mild odor. I had to be sweating again. I hoped she couldn't smell me. My list. My questions. I started to ask them.

There was no past medical history. They were Christian Scientists, had been all their lives. Neither of them had ever been to see a doctor. No hospitalizations. No medications. No physical exams. And she told me, no medical insurance. No hospitalization. No Blue Cross. No Blue Shield. They were paying for this themselves.

So much for past history.

"What happened to him?" I asked.

"He just sort of lapsed into a coma."

"When?"

"Two weeks ago."

"Two weeks!" I was flabbergasted.

"Two weeks ago," she repeated.

"What have you been doing?"

"We," she said firmly, "were praying over him."

"Praying!"

"Of course."

18

"Then why. . . ."

"His brother insisted. I hope I did the right thing."

It was time to examine him. I asked Mrs. Hartung to step outside for a few minutes. The moment of truth was about to start. I could feel my heart rate accelerating. And the sweat building up. My own smell was attacking my nostrils. At least it wouldn't offend Mr. Hartung. He was comatose. I needed a shower in the worst way.

Mrs. Hartung walked over to the bed, took Mr. Hartung's right hand in her two hands, bowed her head and prayed for several minutes, then put his hand back down and turned and left the room.

I was alone with my patient.

Where to start?

The head.

Was there any evidence of trauma?

But there couldn't be. He'd just slowly lapsed into coma. No one had bonked him over the head. Mrs. Hartung had told me he'd just lapsed into a coma. Unless she'd lied to me. Maybe she was the one who'd hit him? Just because they didn't have health insurance didn't mean he didn't have life insurance. After all, she didn't want him to see a doctor. It had been his brother who insisted.

I started at the top. His skull was normal. No bruises. No blood. No evidence of any injury.

Maybe she'd poisoned him.

On to the eyes. Normal color. Normal pupils.

Mouth.

Tongue.

Neck.

Chest.

And so forth.

All the time, my own heart was pounding away. Thank God he was in coma. I was certain the nurse could smell me all the way down the hall at the nursing station.

I was done. I'd found nothing. I pulled out my list. I went over it. I'd done everything, everything I'd written down, and found nothing. I had no idea at all what was wrong with him. Maybe my list was wrong. I'd left something out; I'd forgotten something.

But what?

I had no idea.

William Hartung was comatose and I hadn't figured out the cause. I sat down. I had to think. I couldn't think in there. The smell of my own defeated body filled the room. It was choking me. I needed

19

fresh air. I needed to reread French's.

I got up and left the room. Mrs. Hartung was there waiting for me.

"Doctor," she began, "what's wrong with my husband? Can you help him?"

"I'll be back in a minute," I said and fled down the hall and into the interns' room, locking the door behind me. The room had no windows. Just one narrow cot, a small desk with one lamp, one wooden chair, and one book. French's *Differential Diagnosis,* just as I had left it.

The room was stuffy, but at least it wasn't filled with the odor of my defeat. Not yet, at least. But at the rate I was sweating that wouldn't take very long.

I went over the tables. There had to be something I'd missed, something I'd forgotten, something I could still do.

I couldn't find anything.

Maybe I'd just done a lousy job. That was it. I'd missed something. I'd been too anxious, too nervous. It wasn't that I hadn't done something. It was that I hadn't done something correctly. I had to do it over again.

Back to 1123.

Back to the top of my list.

Back to the smell of my own body.

What smell?

There wasn't any smell in the room, a room that had no ventilation at all. This overheated undersized broom closet had no smell.

It wasn't me. It was him. The odor came from William Hartung, not from Harold Klawans. And it wasn't the smell of defeat. It was the odor of victory.

The musty smell of uremia.

Kidney failure.

I knew what was wrong.

I walked back to 1123. Mrs. Hartung was still there. She once again asked the same two questions.

"What's wrong with my husband? Can you help him?"

"Of course," I said. "Your husband has kidney failure."

The blood tests all confirmed that my diagnosis was correct. William Hartung was in coma because his kidneys had failed, but why had they failed and what could we do about it?

This was 1962, not 1992. We had very few options. Chronic hemodialysis was not in existence. Nor kidney transplants. Not even chronic peritoneal dialysis. But we could do acute peritoneal dialysis, and we were the only hospital in Chicago that could. We had one peritoneal dialysis machine. We could dialyze Mr. Hartung every day until we cleared all the toxins from his system. Then he should wake up, come back from the dead. A twentieth-century Lazarus. Then we could biopsy his kidney. Hopefully we'd find evidence of an acute kidney disease that we could treat. Then we'd treat him and send him home a healthy man. Unless the biopsy showed chronic end-stage kidney disease. Then there would be nothing we could do to treat him. Then we'd stop the dialysis and he'd lapse back into coma and die. Lazarus, too, had eventually died.

We told Mrs. Hartung what we were planning to do. She prayed it would work. And work quickly.

"Why quickly?" the resident asked.

"They have no insurance," I said.

The dialysis worked, and by the fourth day William Hartung was no longer comatose. He was still very lethargic, but he could be aroused. He looked at you when you called his name.

By day six, he was talking, albeit his speech was slurred.

On day ten, his speech was no longer slurred. He could sit up and eat. No more IVs. No more tube feedings. On day fourteen, he was telling jokes. By day twenty-seven, the kidney tests were close enough to normal that we could carry out the biopsy on day twenty-eight. The pathology report came back on day thirty-one.

End-stage chronic renal disease.

There was nothing to do. No acute disease to treat. No infection. No inflammation. No immune response. Nothing. Just chronic end-stage kidney failure.

We could not help him.

And there were other patients who needed the only dialysis unit in town.

Day thirty-seven was his last dialysis.

By day forty-four, he lost his appetite.

On day fifty-two, his speech became slurred, and on day sixty-four, he lapsed back into coma.

William Hartung died on his seventy-ninth day in the hospital. I don't know what the total hospital bill was. I do know that it had reached ten thousand dollars by day twenty-five, and that Mrs. Hartung had tried to get a second mortgage at that point.

I was convinced that the Hartung family would have been better off if they'd stayed in Wisconsin and prayed for a few more days.

21

What good had we done them?

Their life savings were gone. The hope we'd given them turned out to be a false hope.

Mrs. Hartung had had to watch him go into coma twice. Die twice. The first time she had the consolation of prayer. We even robbed her of that.

Two weeks later, I got a note from her, thanking me for all my efforts and for the added few weeks. It had been a wonderful gift. Her prayers had been answered. She and Bill had gotten to be together to talk, to re-share their lives. She would always thank us for that. And God, whose instrument we'd been.

Had Lazarus' wife felt the same way, I wondered?

2

THE GREAT WHITE WHALE

I was rereading Moby Dick *the other day . . . . It's about this whale.*

From *Wonderful Town*
Book and lyrics by
Adolph Comden and Betty Green

Moby Dick. The Great White Whale. Antagonist of Herman Melville's crowning achievement. The single best-known symbol in all nineteenth-century American literature. Moby Dick, pursued across the seas by Ahab, Ishmael, and the rest of the crew of the Pequod.

A great white whale once entered my life. Her name was not Moby Dick; it was Leroux, Harriet Leroux. I did not pursue her across seven seas. I was in no position to pursue anything or anyone. I was an intern, not a sailor. My only harpoons were the five-inch needles we had to use from time to time to perform lumbar punctures (spinal taps) in patients whose extra-thick layers of fat prevented us from using the regular three-inch needles. Harriet Leroux was that fat. She was only twenty-four years old and she was enormously fat, with a severe anemia that accentuated her normal pallor, hence her nickname, The Great White Whale.

Harriet had not always been that fat. She was not one of those fat babies who developed through stages of ever-increasing obesity. Her birth weight had been normal. She had had an average body weight during childhood and adolescence. I saw pictures of her; her father showed them to me more than once. Pictures of his pretty little girl. For some two months she was my patient and I was her intern. We were inexorably linked by whatever fates control such interactions. Our lives became intertwined the day I started my rotation on the Surgical Intensive Care Unit, fondly referred to by its acronym as the SICU. Harriet was a patient there. In fact, she was far more than a patient, she was almost an institution. She'd been in SICU for almost as long as I'd been an intern and undoubtedly she would be there long after I completed my stint. She never got sick enough to die and somehow never got well enough to be transferred to a regular hospital room.

Why did we call her The Great White Whale? Why did we call her anything? On paper her nickname seems almost cruel, and we didn't mean to be cruel. No one ever said it where she could hear. Being in that SICU, as a young doctor, was harrowing. Not just because the patients were so sick, but also because they came and went so quickly. In one day and out the next. I never really knew them. They'd come to us after surgery and leave when they were well enough to recover. I'd know their EKGs, the numbers that came back from the lab, their blood counts, their drugs, but not them. Their histories were what I read in their charts.

Harriet I got to know. She was not just another set of numbers to keep in order. She was our White Whale, a whale we had to protect.

Harriet had ulcerative colitis. She'd had it since she was twelve or thirteen. Her father could tell you every detail of her disease, but those were not the details I needed to do my part to help take care of her. They no longer served any purpose. The diagnosis was not in doubt. Besides, I was not her physician; I was her intern. As such, I had a different, more limited role. It was my job as intern on SICU to keep patients alive. No one was there who did not have a life-threatening disease. All twelve beds were occupied by patients whose lives were in danger, immediate danger, from heart disease, surgical shock, metabolic imbalances, severe infections. Twelve sick patients and two interns who shared the burden. Twenty-four hours on and then twenty-four hours off. My job was to keep them all alive for another twenty-four hours. Understanding Harriet was not within my bailiwick. I looked at the pictures, I listened to the reminiscences, I sat through the stories. But not to see or hear; more to catch my breath. As respite between worries about livers that were failing too much and aortic valves that were leaking too much and kidneys that were not putting out enough urine or too much or losing too much sodium or too much potassium or both.

"Wasn't she a beautiful baby?"

I nodded. I smiled. She had been a pretty little girl.

"Here she is in the first grade."

Second grade. Third. She had been a cute kid. In a tutu, as a ballet student. She was twelve them and moving from cute to more than cute.

24

Age thirteen. The pictures changed. Not the composition. They were still your average home snapshots with jumbled backgrounds and a definite tendency toward silhouetting. The subject looked different. Harriet the sprightly teenager was becoming Harriet the patient. She was thinner, almost gaunt. And paler, much paler. There was no doubt in my mind; she was already sick. Her ulcerative colitis with blood loss resulting in both weight loss and anemia was already well established. She had the unhealthy pallor of Victorian beauties.

I looked at my watch. The patient with a leaky aortic valve and liver failure, I had to check him. And the woman with six kids and no kidney function. Back to work.

The outline of her disease was simple enough and had been repeated over and over in her chart by interns, residents, attending physicians, consultants, surgeons, internists. It had become reduced to a formula, almost a mantra. A life in a series of short phases. A medical litany. The same opening declarative gambit. UGH until twelve—usual good health until she was twelve years old. So much for health. On to disease. The plot thickened. Intermittent melena, black, tarry stools, a sign of bleeding into the gastrointestinal tract. Bloody stools. Diarrhea. Ulcerative colitis diagnosed by proctoscopic examination at age thirteen. UGH was gone forever, a memory along with that vibrant, healthy twelve-year-old in a tutu becoming glowingly pubescent.

Intractable diarrhea.

Weight loss.

More blood loss.

Anemia.

Steroids.

Weight gain.

She became plump, more than plump. And as she did, she got more and more steroids. Whenever they were stopped the diarrhea and bleeding recurred.

More steroids.

More weight. Plump became fat. More than just fat; obese. Harriet was no longer a cute little girl. She had become The Great White Whale, all due to steroids she'd been on for years.

Then the steroids lost their effectiveness. her diarrhea recurred. And with that more bleeding and blood loss. Nothing seemed to work. There were very few other options. She had a bowel that needed to go. Surgery. Removal of the diseased colon, the site of all her misery. Then she could be taken off steroids and live a healthier, better life.

Unfortunately the surgery did not go well, not well at all. Her bowel was too thin to touch, too fragile to cut, too weak to remove. The surgeons had no choice but to patch up the bowel as well as they could and get out.

And so The Great White Whale took up residence in the SICU. Her life there was stormy, a series of complications.

Infections.

Antibiotics.

More steroids.

More infections.

More antibiotics.

More weight gain.

More pallor.

Had Moby Dick been this pale?

She'd get better for a while, not well enough to be discharged but almost. And then she'd have a setback. So she became an institution, a permanent resident in the SICU with the thickest chart in the hospital. That's where I came in. What difference did her distant past make? It was a mere prologue. I had to deal with the present. And that present had more than enough problems of its own. The steroids were all that kept her bowel from dissolving into nothingness, but at the same time, they were suppressing her immune system in a way that we couldn't even measure in 1962. But we could measure the results. Infections, infections everywhere. Abscesses. Some responded to antibiotics. Those that didn't needed to be drained surgically. But only if we could not drain them with a needle, a long needle, one of our own harpoons.

She also had anemia, severe anemia, and thin skin that broke down under pressure, the pressure of her own obesity.

But her infections were becoming less frequent, her anemia less severe, the need for steroids less marked. Hope, it seemed, was just around the corner.

It was Sunday morning. I had worked Saturday. The other intern came in as scheduled at seven-thirty. Together we made rounds and I brought him up to date on our twelve patients; then they were his, all his, until Monday morning. It had been a hectic twenty-four hours. Three deaths. Three new admissions. No one seemed to have gotten any better. Some days were like that. Too many.

"You're down two," was all he said.

I knew just what he meant. I had lost two more patients than he had. I was down two. Eleven to nine.

I went downstairs to the coffee shop. I had not slept a wink in twenty-six hours. I needed sleep and a shave and a shower, and breakfast. The last required the least effort. Halfway through my third cup of coffee and my second toasted bagel with cream cheese, Mr. Leroux sat down next to me. He needed to talk to someone.

I was off duty. I was not his daughter's real doctor. I was an intern. I was exhausted. I was about to beg off when he added, "None of the others will listen to me. They don't want to understand. I know what's wrong. I know how to save my little girl's life."

Saving her life was my business. "Sit down and tell me," I said. He needed a friend. Harriet had other doctors, doctors who knew more about her disease than I did. Maybe I couldn't help, but I could listen.

"It's the water," he confided.

"The water?" I inquired, sipping my cup of coffee.

"The water," he replied confidently. "The water you are drinking. The water from Lake Michigan. With all those chemicals in it. That's what's killing my little girl."

I put down the coffee and turned my attention to the last two bites of bagel.

The story he started to rattle off was simple enough and straightforward enough and clear enough and replete with confirmatory data, far more data than one could have ever imagined, much less asked for. The data went back to age two.

"I thought she was okay until she was twelve," I offered, recalling the introductory phrase of her mantra as well as the cycle of pictures. UGH in a tutu.

At two her mother had died. Of what I never asked and was never told. It was then that the father took charge of little Harriet and her health. She seemed healthy, but was she? Her pediatrician thought so; Mr. Leroux was not so certain. After all she was not regular.

Not regular?

Not at all. Some days she had no bowel movements. Some days two. Occasionally three. What followed amazed me. Mr Leroux could, it seems. recall virtually each bowel movement of his daughter's life in glowing detail.

When Harriet was twelve, they moved to Chicago and the water of Lake Michigan. Disaster struck. Diarrhea. Bloody stools. Watery stools. The history of a patient with severe ulcerative colitis. His story now coincided with the story I already knew far too well. Steroids. Weight gain. Anemia. The Great White Whale. Moby Dick of Lake Michigan. More diarrhea. More blood. Greater and whiter than ever.

Then to my amazement Mr. Leroux produced a series of charts of his own design. His meticulously constructed tables were as well organized as those in the *New England Journal of Medicine.* There were charts of the day-to-day life of Harriet Leroux. These complicated charts plotted the frequency of bowel movements on the abscicca against a variety of variables including fluid consumption and water consumption. Lake Michigan water consumption.

I yearned for another cup of coffee made of that same water. I was tired. My attention was flagging. I wanted to hear what he had to say but what was his point?

It was time for her to go to college. She stayed in the Chicago area. Her father was here. Her doctors. With her medical problem it was far safer to stay near home. She enrolled at Northwestern. More Lake Michigan water. More diarrhea. More charts. More steroids. She was becoming the whale I knew so well.

It was her junior year. All her classmates and friends were going abroad to various European universities in London, Rome, Brussels. She wanted to do the same.

But she was too sick.

She insisted. She was twenty-one and had never stayed anywhere but her own house.

They struck a compromise. She would go to Paris and stay with his sister and go to the University of Paris. So off she went for one year in Paris. It was the best year of her life. The healthiest. No diarrhea. No blood in her stools. She was still not perfectly regular, but better than she'd been in over a decade. She slowly reduced her steroids. She lost weight and was less anemic. She regained some color in her face.

By March she was off steroids. Healthy. Irregular, but healthy.

The year ended. She came back home. She wanted to start ballet classes again.

Home. Chicago. Lake Michigan. Increased irregularity. Increased frequency of stools. It was all there on his charts. Diarrhea. Blood. Bloody stools. He had another table, another chart—too many charts. Anemia. Steroids. More tables, more charts. All documented.

The return of The Great White Whale.

He stopped.

"The water?" I asked.

To him, it was obvious. In Paris, the water did not come from Lake Michigan. It was the water.

The solution.

New water. French bottled water which Harriet had drunk in France. Bottles of Evian water for breakfast, lunch, and dinner. Even the coffee was made from pure, bottled water. He was a man ahead of his time.

Had he tried to give her Evian in the last two years?

Of course.

Had it helped?

He was certain it had. They started with Evian at meals and she improved.

"How much?" I asked.

More charts and more descriptions of each of her bowel movements.

"But she got worse," I objected.

"She brushed her teeth with tap water."

More charts he constructed from his own detailed observations.

Another failure: she bathed in water from Lake Michigan; she showered in it.

There was no stopping him. "But she's on IVs now. She doesn't drink any water."

"Who makes the IV solutions?"

"Baxter Labs."

"Where are they located?"

"Right here, in Chicago. On Lake Michigan."

"Aha!" he triumphed, producing one last chart, comparing frequency and volume of diarrhea versus IV fluid intake. He was convinced that it proved that the more IV fluid we gave her, the worse her diarrhea was.

He had it all backwards of course. When she had more diarrhea, we gave her more fluids. That was how we kept her in balance.

His solution?

IV fluids from France. But the hospital was being obstinate.

Why?

Those fluids weren't approved by the FDA. The administrators said that their hands were tied.

He was in touch with his senator. His senator was sympathetic, but it might take months. He didn't want to waste more months. Nor did Harriet. Would I help?

How?

If he got the IV fluid, would I switch the labels?

I hesitated. It was illegal, but what harm would it do?

None.

"I knew you would."

I had not agreed. I had merely shrugged my shoulders. A friendly shrug. More a gesture of concern than assent.

The IV fluid never came from France and The Great White Whale died. Her death surprised no one. An infection in a patient chronically on steroids can easily get out of control and overwhelm the patient. So it was no surprise, but none of us had really expected it. She was part of the SICU, almost one of the team. She died my last day on SICU. She became my last death during my two months there.

Mr. Leroux still blames the water. He is a prominent environmentalist, on a crusade to clean up the waters of the United States. It won't bring her back. Nothing can do that, but at least some good came from her life.

Harriet Leroux died toward the end of February 1963, in the heyday of Freudian interpretation of life and disease. Psychoanalysis explained it all to everyone bringing together literature (Oedipus) and medicine. One of the diseases it explained was ulcerative colitus. It was all due to developmental arrest in the anal phase. The patients were all anal-retentive or anal-expulsive or both. The Lerouxs fit right in ever so neatly. Harriet's story was the first clinical tale I ever told from beginning to end to friends. Everyone understood all of its neat Freudian implications, implications far too blunt to be subtle interpretations. Then I stopped telling it. It was far too neat, far too obvious, and I was becoming more and more skeptical of such obvious explanations. I stopped long before Freud-bashing became popular.

Today analysis is out even in Chicago, which has long been one of its major bastions. Freudian views of causation no longer ring true. The abused little girls, whom Freud treated as adults, had not fantasized; they'd been molested. Harriet's story is no longer the same story. It no longer conveys the message it once so readily conveyed. Her father's obsessive attention didn't cause her ulcerative colitis.

Ulcerative colitis is a real disease, now classified as autoimmune. We now believe that for some reason Harriet's immune system was producing antibodies that attacked her bowel. That's why the steroids helped her: They suppressed the production of those deadly antibodies. Her father merely recorded these abnormalities.

I began to tell Harriet's story again, and her father's story, from beginning to end even though it has nothing to do with neurology. Why? Probably because I think about patients and their diseases far differently than I once did.

And perhaps it isn't either—or, Freudian or autoimmune. Maybe the two are not mutually exclusive.

What triggers an autoimmune response?

What focused Harriet's antibodies on her bowel? What precipitated her attacks?

It sure as hell wasn't Chicago's drinking water.

3

CURRENT OF INJURY

If you really want to advise me, do it on Saturday afternoon between one and four o'clock. And you've got twenty-five seconds to do it, between plays. Not on Monday. I know the right thing to do on Monday.

Alex Agase
University of Michigan
assistant football coach

William Marshall was the fourteenth patient with an acute myocardial infarction who had been admitted to my care during my internship. He was admitted in early April, my sixth month on one of the acute medical services. He had had the onset of crushing chest pain and severe shortness of breath while running from his office to the train—a mad dash he made almost every day to catch the 5:45 express in order to be home for dinner at 6:30. It represented most of the exercise he ever got, unless you counted his occasional stroll over to court, but as a senior partner in a law firm that specialized in patent law, that only happened once or twice a year. His heart attack had stopped him in his tracks at 5:30.

He arrived in our Emergency Room at 6:13.

The doctors in the ER gave him some morphine, hooked him up to an oxygen mask, started an IV, and shipped him up to me. All in less than ten minutes.

Those were the days before cardiac monitoring. We had no monitors, no Medical Intensive Care Unit, no specific Coronary Care Unit. We had general medical floors and patients with heart attacks were admitted to these floors. That was why William Marshall was sent to me.

He got to my floor at 6:30, just as his wife was deciding that he had missed his train again. She would feed the kids and have dinner with him at 7:15. After checking to see that his pulse and blood pressure were still stable, I took his history.

He was fifty-two years old.

He was a heavy cigarette smoker and had been for over thirty years. He smoked a pack and a half a day. Today we would make a simple calculation and categorize him as having forty-five pack years of self-immolation. Then, we just knew smoking was bad even without knowing all the details.

He had mild hypertension but was on no treatment for it.

And his dad had died of a heart attack.

In short, William Marshall had most of the risk factors for an MI: smoking, high blood pressure, and a positive family history.

I examined him. His blood pressure was still slightly elevated, 155/100. His pulse was normal, both its rate and its rhythm. There was nothing much of note on the rest of his exam.

His pain had been relieved by the morphine. That was a good sign—or at least better than the bad sign of pain that did not respond to morphine. His oxygen was running. So was his IV. There was only one more thing to do; run an EKG. That was one of my tasks. I went to the nursing station where the EKG machine was kept, atop the acute coronary care cart (the so-called crash cart), and wheeled the entire cart back to Mr. Marshall's room. I attached the electrodes, one to each wrist, one to the left ankle, and one to his chest and flicked on the machine and watched the strip of EKG paper roll out of the machine.

There was no question about it. He'd had an MI. The evidence of damage was right there on the EKG. It demonstrated his acute injury. What the cardiologists called a "current of injury." And he had a big current of injury, as big as any I'd ever seen. It distorted the shape of each and every heartbeat being recorded by the EKG.

One more strip and I'd be done. And on to my next patient. All I needed was a long rhythm strip to check the rhythm of the heartbeats, not the shape of each individual beat.

I switched the appropriate switch and flicked the machine back on.

His rhythm was normal, even regular. A normal sinus rhythm, driven by the sinus node—the heart's normal pacemaker. When the heart is injured, the walls of the ventricle become irritated and can set up alternative pacemakers which initiate abnormal beats or rhythms. A single abnormal beat is called a premature ventricular contraction (PVC), a pair bigeminy, a triplet trigeminy; bursts are now called salvos, and a continuous run is called ventricular tachycardia (V-tach). The latter is an ominous sign often ending up as continuous wriggling/fluttering of the heart wall in which no blood is pumped—ventricular fibrillation or V-fib, a state that unless quickly reversed by defibrillation is uniformly fatal.

William Marshall's rhythm looked fine. Normal sinus rhythm. No PVCs. No arrythmias at all.

So much for his EKG.

I reached over to switch off the EKG machine. Right before my very eyes, the rhythm changed. Gone was the normal heart rhythm. The heats had become markedly abnormal. Not just PVCs, or bigeminy or trigeminy. Not merely a salvo of abnormal bursts, but the onset of World War III.

V-tach.

V-fib and death could not be far off.

This was not an emergency. It was close to terror.

The EKG machine was still running and spilling a trail of paper onto the floor, more because I forgot to turn it off than any notion that continuing to monitor his rhythm would prove valuable; after all, continuous monitoring was not something I had ever seen being done. I ignored the paper and searched through the crash cart to find the medicine I wanted. It had to be there somewhere. But where? Then I saw it right where it always was. Pronestyl, known generically as procaine amide. It was the treatment of choice of V-tach. In fact, it was the only treatment. And I had it in my own shaking hand.

I grabbed a syringe.

I had never seen a patient during and episode of V-tach. I had never treated V-tach. But I had been taught what to do.

I drew up the correct dosage—200 milligrams—reached over, and started to inject it into his IV.

Mr. Marshall could feel the pounding in his chest.

"What's wrong?" he asked, obviously frightened.

"The rhythm's a bit too fast," I replied.

I pushed the syringe, and in a flash the Pronestyl had been injected. Not as a slow infusion, but as a single bolus.

I felt his chest.

The V-tach was still there. I could feel it.

Go away, I said to myself.

NOW.

V-Tach.

Unchanged. Pounding against my hand. Against his chest and through his chest wall into my palpating fingers.

Then it began to change. Not every beat was an explosion.

Some were soft, like normal heartbeats.

First one.
Then a pair.
Then three in a row.
Four.
Five.
Six.
All soft. Regular. Normal.

I'd done it. Automatically. I'd seen a V-tach. I'd recognized it. I'd treated it. And Mr. Marshall was alive and well.

At that moment, I knew that my internship had done its job. All those long hours of drudgery. All those nights of continuous stress. The process had worked. I knew how to react to disease, how to make decisions about sick people all by myself. In one way, the one that counted most, there was nothing more to learn.

At that moment, the cardiology fellow walked in. Cardiology had been asked to see Mr. Marshall in consultation.

I told him what had happened.

He seized the growing pile of EKG paper. I didn't even know it was there. I started to apologize for forgetting to turn off the machine and wasting all that paper.

He shushed me. He had an EKG to read.

"V-tach," he said, reading the rhythm strip. "I've never seen a record of what happens when someone goes from V-tach to normal sinus rhythm," he added, then went on to describe the changing rhythms with a wealth of detail I didn't quite understand, "Six to five Wenckebach, four to three, two to one. This is unbelievable. You did a great job."

That night we kept Mr. Marshall attached to the EKG machine and monitored him by running rhythm strips off and on. By morning, his room was filled with piles of used EKG paper, all showing normal sinus rhythm.

The cardiology fellow made copies of the tracings demonstrating the transformation from V-tach to normal. All the cardiologists wanted to study them. That fellow is now a senior attending cardiologist and although monitoring has made such documentation a common experience, he still has his copy of the EKG as part of his files.

I don't. I never did. I was not that interested in cardiology. There was nothing more I could learn from that EKG. It could not become an instrument I would use for teaching. It had been a test to measure what I had already learned.

And I'd passed.

William Marshall survived more than one episode of V-tach. He survived his entire MI. He went home three weeks later, no longer a smoker. In two months he was back at work. I only saw him once more, when his brother had a stroke. He was sixty-four then and had retired. He died a few years later of another MI—his third. He died at home, before the ambulance arrived.

4

THE PHALLUS FROM DALLAS

"Does your dog bite?" The Inspector asked.
"No," the hotelkeeper replied.
The Inspector then tried to pet the dog, which proceeded to bite him.
"I thought you said your dog doesn't bite," the Inspector protested.
"It's not my dog."

Old vaudeville routine appropriated in
The Return of the Pink Panther

He was the head of Obstetrics and Gynecology when I was in medical school and for the life of me I can't recall his name, but I do recall his nickname. We all referred to him as The Phallus from Dallas. He had, it seems, been in Texas somewhere before he came to the University of Illinois. He was universally disliked, on both personal and scientific grounds.

One of the professional reasons he was disliked was his liberal use of blood transfusions for pregnant women. That was long before AIDS, but we knew all about serum hepatitis, an often serious and occasionally fatal infection of the liver caused by a virus and spread by transfusions from apparently healthy donors. And, at that time, there was no way to screen the blood. So each transfusion carried a potential risk.

All surgeons were cautious. Only use blood when you really had to and never give a single transfusion. If that's all the patient needed, that patient was safer without it. The rule was the same on every surgery service:

General surgery. Cancer surgery.

Ear, nose, and throat.

But not OB.

The Phallus had his own rule. If any woman entered labor with a hemoglobin below eleven, she got blood—ONE UNIT.

We were all horrified.

The University of Illinois ran a large clinic for poor, mostly black patients with poor nutritional status. For them, eleven was a normal hemoglobin. And if one of these normal women came in to the University of Illinois for her delivery, she got ONE UNIT of blood and with it a risk of developing serum hepatitis.

We asked him about it. We challenged him.

He sneered his usual sneer. What did we know? We were mere medical students. Third-year students, and not very bright ones at that. He was the Chairman of Obstetrics and Gynecology and he'd been practicing medicine that way—giving one unit of blood prior to delivery to any pregnant woman with a hemoglobin below eleven— and he'd never seen a single one of these women get serum hepatitis. Not one. He was certain that their pregnant state protected them. That and their color.

End of discussion.

My uncle was an obstetrician. I told him the story. He listened to the end and then nodded.

"He's probably right."

"You mean they don't get hepatitis?"

"No. He didn't say that exactly. He said he'd never seen one get hepatitis. And I'm sure he never has."

"So they are immune?"

"Of course not."

"I don't understand," I complained. I was just a confused third-year medical student.

"If you were a young woman with a healthy three- or four-month-old baby, and you turned yellow, would you go to your obstetrician?"

"No. I'd see an internist or go to the nearest Emergency Room."

"So, he's right. He's never seen a case of serum hepatitis in any of the women he gave that unnecessary one unit. Other doctors see them."

The Phallus had not lied to us. Nor had the hotelkeeper lied to the Inspector. It was funnier in the movie.

5

ABSENCE OF RESPIRATION

Absence of respiration is a bad sign.

Apocryphal aphorism
attributed to Hippocrates

*You do not die all at once. Some tissues live on for minutes, even hours,
giving still their little cellular shrieks, molecular echoes of the agony of
the whole corpus.*

Richard Selzer, MD

William Jessup was not the first patient whose death I witnessed, nor the last. But he was the first patient for whose death I
was no more than a witness. I had participated in scenes of death,
sometimes quite actively: breathing into a mouth I had never seen
before, pounding on an unfamiliar chest, squeezing blood into an
anonymous IV line. Sometimes not quite so actively: scanning a cardiac monitor, drawing up medications, relaying orders. But never as
a witness only. It was not a role with which I was at all comfortable.

All of the frantic scenes of CPR, of emergency surgery, of controlled panic, have congealed into one amorphous memory. They
have become an experience, a rite of passage, an obstacle course
without name, without identity and without passion.

Not so William Jessup. I remember his name, his diagnosis, his
death, my helplessness, my thoughts, and my role as final witness.

The moment I entered his room that evening I knew what was
expected of me. I had been anticipating this. I had hoped it would
happen when someone else was on duty, one of the neurosurgeons.
He was really their patient, not mine. We had a combined neurology-
neurosurgery service and we alternated coverage. That night I was
on call for both Neurology and Neurosurgery, and that was the night
when William Jessup was going to die.

I looked at our patient and wondered how I could get through the next ten minutes. Ten minutes of doing nothing, of prolonging no agonies. Of letting nature take its course.

I tried to keep my mind occupied. Tried to think of something else. Something other than a man dying of a brian tumor. A man who a mere five months earlier had been leading a full, active, normal life. Father. Husband. Engineer. Little League coach. Owner of a small bungalow, a beat-up station wagon, an expanding brain tumor.

There had to be something else to think about. Something. Someone.

George Gershwin. His name burst into my consciousness and could not be suppressed. And I knew why.

This had to have been how George Gershwin had died—and countless others over the centuries. For, like George Gershwin, William Jessup had had a malignant brain tumor. In 1938, there had really been nothing to do for Gershwin. In 1968, when I walked into Mr. Jessup's hospital room, there was nothing more that I could do. He'd already had a course of radiation therapy that had added a couple of months to his life. No more than that. Today, we would also administer steroids and chemotherapy, but the outlook for patients with rapidly growing malignant brain tumors, glioblastomas, isn't all that much better despite all our hopes and efforts.

I knew what to do and what not to do. And I would do it. Not the nurse. Me. Not the family. They were at home. I'd call them later. They had already said their goodbyes, and he could no longer hear them. I told the nurse who had called me in to see the patient to leave the room. She did. And then I was alone with my patient and his brain tumor.

Had Gershwin died alone? Or had his family been at his bedside? His brother Ira? Did it matter?

The words of Gershwin's last completed song started to sing itself in my brain.

No, I reminded myself. Those were not George Gershwin's last words. The last song completed by the brothers Gershwin was entitled "Our Love Is Here to Stay." There was nothing prophetic, neither the title nor the words. George had not written them as his ironic farewell. He never wrote the words; he only wrote those wonderful, indestructible melodies. His older brother, Ira, had written those words, as he wrote the words to almost every song that George composed. Ira went on to live another forty years, and to write hundreds of other song lyrics for a half a dozen different composers.

My rendition of the song ended. I was left with only the sound of my own breathing, for William Jessup was now no longer breathing. That was why I had been summoned into his room. His breathing had become shallow, irregular, erratic, agonal, and now it was gone. Absence of respiration. All I had to do was wait a couple of minutes longer. Three or four at the most. For that is how patients with brain tumors die. The tumor expands. The brain swells. The brain stem, which controls respiration, becomes displaced by the swelling. Displaced, stretched and distorted. And those delicate structures of the brain stem that control respiration become compromised.

Respiration stops.

Once respiration ceases the oxygen content of the blood tumbles. The heart, deprived of oxygen, soon crumbles and fails. It only takes a few minutes, five or six at the most. All I had to do was stand around for those five or six minutes thinking of Gershwin tunes. It seemed like an eternity.

It never occurred to me to place William Jessup on a respirator—or, more correctly, a ventilator. Ventilators do not breathe or respire for the patient, they merely ventilate the patient—move air in and out of his lungs. And that was just what his brain was no longer telling his diaphragm and the respiratory muscles to do. It was in that sense a simple mechanical failure. The thought of overcoming that physical failure never crossed my mind.

Good air was not coming in. Bad air was not going out. His muscles were immobile. A simple ventilator could overcome all that.

In with the good air.

Out with the bad air.

But to what end? Putting him on such ventilation would only serve to prolong his agonal state—his process of dying. Not his agony. He was already unconscious, comatose. A ventilator would not change that. The reticular activating system of the brain stem controls consciousness. It and the respiratory centers co-mingle. His reticular system was stretched, distorted, and displaced and was no longer activating the rest of his brain. As a result he was in coma; his conscious agony was over.

I tried to think of other Gershwin lyrics, written by Ira to the tunes of composers other than George. Nothing came to me.

I put my stethoscope on William Jessup's chest.

There was no sound of air rushing in and out to mask the sounds of his heart. Those heart sounds were all that was left. Good old lub and dub, thumping away as if nothing had happened.

I lifted my stethoscope. It remained dangling from my ears.

43

Ira Gershwin.

Kurt Weill.

Lady in the Dark.

"I love Russian Composers." The names of fifty-one Russian composers sung in fifty-three seconds by Danny Kaye. The only names I could come up with were Mussorgsky and Shostakovich.

I listened again.

The sounds were still there.

Fainter. But still there. And still regular.

Lub-dub. Lub-dub. Lub-dub . . . .

Then the end began.

Lub . . . . . dup. Lub lub . . . . . Lub.

And once it began, it did not take long. I waited.

I listened.

I heard the last lub. And then listened on. To nothing.

I went out of the room and nodded to the nurse.

She nodded back.

William Jessup was dead.

Just like George Gershwin.

I could have done something. I could have delayed the inevitable. He could have lived longer.

Days longer, weeks, months.

So could Gershwin. But there would have been no more songs, no more melodies.

I knew that night that I had done the right thing, the only responsible thing. I could have put him on a respirator, but then I would have had to turn it off. I or someone else. And turning it off would be an active step. A step involved in legal and ethical conundrums, such as the termination of medical care, withdrawal of life-saving support, withdrawal of life itself.

Give me a break.

Give George Gershwin a break.

Let him die in peace.

What if someone with a different sort of compassion had put William Jessup on a ventilator that night?

Or George Gershwin thirty years earlier. It's a bit of an anachronism I know, but think about the possibility. A ventilator with a life of its own and a brain tumor that eats of the brain but rarely enters the body.

A LATE COMPLICATION

Emil Michaels came under my care for only a short time and he was never exactly my patient, but as a result of one of those peculiarities of scheduling, his death and my life became inexorably linked. Emil was forty-seven at the time. He had had severe neurologic problems for over a dozen years, ever since he had been hit by a drunken driver while standing at a bus stop waiting for a bus. The car, which swerved off the road without braking, hit Emil and threw him into a wall, breaking his back. The displaced vertebra, in turn, crushed Emil's spinal cord and left him a paraplegic, paralyzed from the waist down.

That had all happened in 1955. I met Emil in 1967. He had come into the hospital because he was running a high fever as a result of another in a long series of urinary-tract infections. These were a direct complication of his spinal-cord injury. Because of the injury, he could not control his bladder and required a permanent catheter. Such catheters almost always become infected sooner or later, and when they do, the infections are often recurrent and difficult to treat, much less cure. That was the case with Emil Michaels. He had daily temperature spikes of 104 degrees and the infection had reached his kidneys. He had been admitted to the Internal Medicine Service, and Neurology was asked to see him in consultation in order to evaluate his neurologic condition.

I was the senior resident in Neurology at the time and one of my duties was to see all of the neurologic consultations in the hospital. Emil was one of the four consults I was asked to see that evening. As far as I could tell, he would be the least interesting of the four. I cannot remember why I was asked to see the other three. In fact, I have no recall of them at all, but very few neurologic problems are less exciting that the unchanging status of a patient with an old, stable paraplegia. I triaged Emil to the bottom of my list and finally got to see him around eleven-thirty, after my other three consults and a couple of short unscheduled trips to the emergency room.

I can still picture him. He was seated in bed, reading. His fever had broken so he was no longer uncomfortable. He had a full head of dark hair. In those days, few men of his age wore their hair long. He did. Not long enough to comb into a pony-tail, but long enough to look like an unruly mane. He did not look up from his book.

I introduced myself.

He put down the book and without hesitating said "T-nine crush injury with a resulting L-one level."

In everyday English that meant that his ninth thoracic verte-bra (the ninth of those vertebra that give off ribs that surround our lungs) had been crushed, resulting in severe damage to the spinal cord that it's supposed to protect. The spinal cord is arranged lon-gitudinally. Those segments that serve the neck and arms are clos-est to the brain, but the cord is shorter than the spine so that a T-9 level does not cause loss of function from T-9 down, but "only" from about L-1 or L-2, the base of the abdomen, the groin, and below.

"Complete loss?" I asked, since it appeared that he understood the lingo.

"Motor, bladder, sensory, everything," he nodded.

"All modalities of sensation?" Outside the spinal cord, the nerves each carry all the different types of sensory experience, but once they enter the spinal cord, all that changes. Different classes or modalities of sensation are carried by different tracts or pathways within the spinal cord. Pain and temperature share one, touch another, position sense a third, and so forth. Because of this arrange-ment, an injury to the spinal cord, if incomplete—that is, if only a part of the cord is involved—can affect one type of sensation more than others or even spare one while devastating the others.

"The whole ball of wax."

It was late. There was another patient waiting in the ER and someone else I wanted to check once more in the ICU before I went to bed. Should I even bother to examine him? He'd had an old T-9 fracture with an L-2 level. He knew it. He'd already told me what the results of my examination of him would be.

Why bother him?

Why waste my time?

We both had better things to do.

But this was what I was supposed to do, so I did it: I examined him from top to bottom. First his motor exam, then his sensory exam. The motor exam revealed just what I expected; he was intact above L-2 and completely paralyzed below that level. The sensory examination didn't. He should have had normal sensation to all modalities above the L-2 and total absence of all sensation below that level: the whole ball of wax. But that wasn't what I'd found. The loss below L-2 was complete. He'd been right about that. The injury to his cord had been complete. Everything was lost below it. Touch, pain (tested with a sharp pin and known in medication circles as pinprick sensation), temperature, position sense, and even vibratory sensation tested with a tuning fork.

Emil had been right about that.

But he wasn't entirely normal above L-2. Pretty good, but not normal. Touch was fine. So were position sense and vibration, but not pain and temperature; they were lost all the way up to his neck. That gave him a pinprick level of about T-1 up to the top thoracic segment of his spinal cord, that was over a foot away from the L-2 segment.

This was most unusual. This pattern of sensory findings in which pain and temperature are severely impaired and all else is spared is known as dissociated sensory loss. It is only seen in disorders of the spinal cord and is made possible by the fact that the nerve fibers that carry different modalities of sensation segregate together and form separate pathways or tracts within the spinal cord. The tract for both pain and temperature follow a special course. These fibers cut across to the outside of the cord before they start heading up toward the brain and are known as crossed fibers: They have crossed within the spinal cord. The ones for position and vibration stay on the same side of the cord (uncrossed), while touch itself is converged by both crossed and uncrossed fibers. Either group of fibers, if working, is sufficient to relay the appropriate messages.

Emil had lost pinprick and temperature. Everything else was fine. That meant that some process had attacked the fibers carrying these sensations within the spinal cord and left the other fibers alone.

But where? And what?

The where was easy. That happened only in one place: right in the center of the spinal cord. That's where the fibers crossed, in the center of the cord, both those from the right carrying pain and temperature from the right side of the body and those from the left carrying the same sensations from the left side of the body. Emil had lost pain and temperature from both sides of his body equally. That meant that whatever had caused this had interrupted the pain and temperature fibers at the exact point where the pathways from the two sides of the body crossed. But not just at one place. The fibers for the T-1 level cross at about T-1, those for L-1, at L-1. He'd lost pain and temperature from T-1 to L-1 or vice versa. That represented about one foot of spinal cord. That meant that something was wrong with Mr. Michael's spinal cord, the exact center of his spinal cord all the way from L-1, just above his old crush injury, to T-1, but that the rest of his spinal cord was working fine between T-1 and L-1. Now what, I wondered, could do that?

Then I realized that I'd examined him all wrong. I'd been so focused on examining him and documenting his unchanging neurologic deficit that I'd neglected to take his history, and history is the single most important factor in making a neurologic diagnosis. It is the history that allows you to interpret your examination, to understand it, to translate the findings into a meaningful pattern that represents not just a set of individual results but a specific disease. That was the interpretation I needed.

"Other than your L-two level," I began, "do you have any other neurologic problem,"

"You know, Doc," he replied, "I do. Why are you asking?"

I explained my dilemma and he in turned explained his symptoms. For the last three or four years he'd noticed that he had some peculiar problems above his old L-2 level. At first, he was worried that the entire level might be changing. Could that happen?

No, I assured him. It couldn't.

He was relieved to hear that.

What had he noticed?

Things felt different. First on his stomach, then his chest, and now all the way up to his neck.

What did he mean by different? Did he still feel everything?

Yes, he still felt everything.

That figured. Touch sensation had been normal to my examination.

But, he explained, the quality was different. Things just didn't feel right.

That was because some of his touch fibers, the crossed ones, were lost. The uncrossed ones allowed him to appreciate the phenomenon of touch, but qualitative interpretation of rough versus smooth requires more than that.

Had he noticed anything else?

He had. He'd also realized that he could no longer tell hot from cold. That, too, had progressed upward over the last few years. As had his ability to feel pain or pinpricks.

Was I certain the whole level wouldn't change?

I was.

How sure? He was worried that his entire body would become dead like his legs. First his stomach, then his chest, then his arms, his neck. Everything. Dead. Numb. Senseless.

No. No. That was not going to happen.

"Are you sure of that?"

I started to reassure him once again, but stopped in midsentence. How could I make such predictions? I had no idea what he had. I had no diagnosis. Without that, prediction was impossible. All predictions are based on an understanding of the usual natural progression of a specific disease. Once you knew what the patient had and knew enough about the natural history of his disease in general so far in that specific patient, you could make predictions. But so far, I was in no position to even hazard a guess, much less give guarantees off the top of my head. And although I was still a resident, I knew that patients heard such reassurances as iron-clad guarantees.

What did he have?

His findings suggested that he had a problem in the center of his cord, from L-2 to T-1. The commonest cause of such a problem was a long, narrow fluid-filled cyst or syrinx. The full diagnostic term is syringomyelia syrinx or tube of the spinal cord. But I'd never heard of a syrinx beginning at L-2. Syrinxes of the cord invariably started in the neck—never anywhere else. His had not only not started in his neck, it hadn't even gotten there. His neck region was completely normal. His problem, whatever it was, started where his spinal cord had been crushed. Crush injuries had nothing to do with syrinxes. Syrinxes started by themselves, as small outpouches of the fine central canal of the spinal cord, not as a result of spinal injury. But Emil Michaels had had a severe spinal injury and whatever he had started at the upper end of that old injury and had been spreading or expanding up from that spot for four or five years. And it sure acted like a syrinx. But was it? And if so, where had it come from? It was hard to imagine that whatever was going on had no relationship at all to his old injury, but I'd never read about a syrinx as a late complication of spinal cord injury. Of course, I was still just a resident. Perhaps one of the more experienced neurologists would be able to make a precise diagnosis.

"Well," he said interrupting my meandering thoughts, "what will happen to me?"

I hesitated.

49

"What's wrong with me?"

"I don't know," I admitted, but I still didn't think he had that much to worry about.

How could I say that, if I didn't even know what was going on?

It was a feeling. No, it was more than a feeling. His problem had stayed in the center of his cord for four years. It had spread upwards, but it had stayed in the center of his cord. It had not gone laterally to involve other tracts. It had not invaded the motor system. I saw no reason to believe that it would change its nature and move laterally instead of up.

"So it may continue to move up my body?"

"It probably will," I granted, "unless we can make a diagnosis and treat it."

"Treat what?"

I didn't know.

Nor did the staff neurologist with whom I discussed Mr. Michaels. He doubted that we'd ever know unless Mr. Michaels died and we managed to obtain an autopsy and the pathologists were conscientious enough to remove the spinal cord, which was no easy feat. Even then . . . .

"But what does he have?"

"Who knows? Sometimes things like this happen to people. And we just don't know. You just have to learn that. We can't always make a diagnosis."

It was not a lesson I had any interest in learning. Not because of any great altruistic desire to help every single patient by making the diagnosis; after all, many diagnoses that neurologists make are of untreatable disease and often the prognoses that can be derived are not very cheerful. No, my need to make a diagnosis sprang from something else, from a need of my own. I went into neurology to be a consulting diagnostician. To solve problems. The nervous system and its myriad pathways and patterns of function were like some giant set of mazes. And each time something went wrong someplace, the involved maze changed, but there was still a way out, a solution, a diagnosis. And I needed to find that diagnosis. That was what I was all about.

"Sometimes things like this happen" was not acceptable. Not to me. Was that merely part of the bravado of youth? A form of neurologic hubris? Would it pass in time? My teachers all thought so.

I went back to see Mr. Michaels the next day. I re-examined him. Nothing had changed on his neurologic examination. I hadn't thought

50

anything would. Whatever progression was going on was far too slow to be measured by daily examinations. I had just wanted to be certain of my findings, to double-check myself. I found the exact same dissociated sensory exam I had found the night before.

He again asked me what was wrong.

I again did not know.

He once more asked what was going to happen to him and I once more told him what I could, based upon what he had told me and my understanding of the mazes of the anatomy of the spinal cord.

He was once more unconcerned. So we talked about André Gide. The book he was reading was a novel by Gide, *Lafcadio's Adventures.* I had read much of Gide. Emil Michaels had never been a great reader, until his injury. And there was only so much TV he could tolerate. He started to read. First thrillers. Then the more literate thrillers, Graham Greene, Eric Ambler, then real novels. His daughter had introduced him to modern French writers, starting with —

"Camus. *The Stranger,*" I guessed.

He was amazed.

It was not an amazing guess. That's the French novel all college kids started with. It was the one I had started with. I had to go.

"Come back tomorrow," he requested.

I said I would. And I did. I saw him every day. Not to re-examine him; I never examined him again during that hospital stay. Nor to talk about his disease. We never did. We talked about literature. But that was not my real reason for these visits. Seeing him forced me to look at him and think again about the problem, my problem.

Not Gide.

Not Camus.

Not Malraux.

Diagnosis.

I even met his daughter one day. We talked of Sartre and Giradoux. And she, too, never asked me about the diagnosis. It was as if that failure was the one subject we had to avoid.

Finally, the antibiotics triumphed. The infection was gone. His urine was free of bacteria. So were his kidneys and bladder. And he was no longer running any fever. So they sent him home. I came around that day to see him and he was gone. No one had notified me that he was leaving. There was no reason to. Medically, I wasn't doing anything but thinking. And that I could do on my own time.

And I did. I devoured every article I could find on spinal-cord injuries, starting with one written by Henry Head, later Sir Henry, in

1915. One of the great names in British neurology and at one time the editor of what was then the most prestigious neurology journal, *Brain,* he studied the spinal cords of British soldiers in the Great War who had died following severe cord injuries. It was a landmark study. The cord, Head pointed out, consisted of two types of tissue that were of quite different consistency. The soft gray part in the center was made up of cells that sent nerves out into the body. The firm outer part was made up of the tracts that carried messages to and from the brain. The anatomic information I already knew—I'd learned that as a first-year medical student—it was the information on consistency that was new and important. In essence, the spinal cord is like a tube of toothpaste. The fiber tracts are like the outer tube itself, the central core like the toothpaste. If you squeeze a tube of toothpaste in the middle, you deform the tube itself, but only at the level you are squeezing. The toothpaste is displaced, pushed upward and downward into that part of the paste that was not part of the original squeeze. And that, according to Head, was what happened in a crush injury to the cord. That intrigued me. It showed how the central part of the cord could be involved about the level of the crush itself, as cord tissue was squeezed and pushed upward right in the center, right where the fibers carrying pain and temperature crossed.

But that all happened at the time of the injury. Why would that start to get worse seven or eight years later? Head was silent on such issues. His patients had all died. They had no antibiotics then.

I read on. Nothing seemed to help. Things such as this may have happened, but no one had written about them. I forged on. I had started with the major journals: *Brain, Neurology, Neurosurgery.* Now I was reading the lesser ones and still coming up empty. Two weeks of such frustration and I gave up. I'd gone through everything and found nothing.

About a month later, I got a phone call. It was Emil's daughter. Her father was worse and he was very worried. I told them to bring him in so I could examine him. He came to the hospital that afternoon and I examined him.

He *was* worse. His loss of sensation had extended to a higher level. It was up to the middle of his neck. It had moved up several more segments of his spinal cord: another two or three inches. His brain was now only a couple of inches away. And he was scared. He asked me the same questions. I gave him the same bad answers.

"Doc, you've got to help me!"

I told him what I'd done, all the journals I'd read. All the books I'd explored. I didn't know what more to do.

"Read more books," he said.

"There aren't any more."

"There are always more books. No one can read them all."

He was right about that. The medical literature, even then, was all but inexhaustible.

"Do it for me, won't you?" he asked.

I would. I'd try again. We tried to talk about something else. He had moved northward and was now reading Scandinavian novels. Pär Lagerkvist. Knut Hamsun. Did I know that Hamsun had once worked in Chicago as a bus driver?

I didn't, and even though that made Hamsun the first Nobel Prize-winning writer to have lived in Chicago or anywhere in the USA, it didn't seem to matter. The feeling of defeat hung over me. I needed to know the answer. Not for him, for me. He had a neurologic disease that was progressing before my own eyes and I knew its precise location in the inside of his spinal cord and its exact dimensions. I could draw it inside a diagram of his spinal cord in all three directions, yet I couldn't name it. What did I care about Knut Hamsun?

He was still talking. Had I read any Hamsun?

He waited, and when I said nothing began talking about Hamsun's greatest novel, *Hunger.* In a couple of minutes, he moved on to Lagerkvist. *The Dwarf, The Sybil, Barabbas.* He named several more. I didn't even hear the titles.

"Hamsun," I said.

"What about him?"

"During the war, during the Nazi occupation of Norway, he was a collaborator. A Nazi? Did you know that?"

He didn't.

The conversation was over. He went home and I made my rounds. Later that week, when I had a couple of free hours, I went once again to the library. There were new patients with other problems that I knew I should read about, new diseases I should have looked up. I started again with spinal-cord injuries, back with World War I and Sir Henry Head. He now seemed an old friend. I was comfortable with his ideas, his descriptions of what happened to the cord during a crush injury. I was comfortable because I already knew what he had written. Rereading it didn't help me or Emil Michaels.

I was sorry I'd said what I had about Knut Hamsun. Not because it wasn't true. It was; he had been a Nazi sympathizer. Not because that was irrelevant. That's never irrelevant, but because of the way I'd said it. Emil had tried to be a friend. I'd cut him to the quick. I'd administered a pain he could feel.

The library had a new book. It was the proceedings of a meeting on spinal-cord injuries, sponsored by the Veterans Administration. World War I had not been the only war that caused spinal-cord injuries. They also occurred in World War II and in the Korean conflict, but with a difference. More victims survived because of better nursing care, better surgical care, and antibiotics; especially because of antibiotics. They survived and ended up in VA hospitals, in special spinal-cord units. And the VA sponsored a meeting on such patients. I looked through the index. The word *syringomyelia* was not there. I read through the table of contents. No mention of it. I skimmed the book from cover to cover.

Another failure.

And this was the latest word, The Thirteenth Veterans Administration Conference on Spinal Cord Injury. If this was the proceedings of number thirteen, there had to be proceedings of the other twelve, but where? Who had them? How could I get them?

I asked the librarian. The library could order them for me, three at a time. It would take about ten days to get them. Which volumes did I want first?

"One, two, and three," I said. I'd start at the beginning.

It took two weeks, but the books came. I could keep them for three days. I took them home with me and each night I went through one of them. I'd start with the index, then the table of contents, then the various papers, one at a time. And each night I found nothing. So three days later I returned them and ordered three more volumes.

"Four, five, and six," I said.

Ten days later they arrived.

Three days later I brought them back, none the wiser, and requested three more. "Seven, eight, and nine."

On the day they were to arrive, Emil Michaels called me.

"Dr. Klawans," he began, "it's Mr. Michaels."

No "Doc." No "Emil."

"You remember me. I'm the one with the spinal cord injury who's getting worse."

Of course I remembered him. I was still living with his disease, whatever it was. I had six more volumes to go. After that, I had no idea what I'd do, but I was still trying. Did I remember him? What a question!

"How are you, Emil?" I asked, being careful to use his first name.

"I'm worse, Dr. Klawans," he replied formally.

"Damn," I replied. Angry at him for getting worse so quickly. I still had six more volumes to read.

"More of me isn't working right, Doctor." Still formal, but less so.

"How high is it now?" I asked.

"My chin," he said.

I could hear his questions being readied. I didn't want to deal with them again until I had a real answer. I had six more volumes to review. That meant six nights of reading and ten days of waiting in between.

"I'll see you in three weeks," I said.

"Don't you want to examine me now?" he pleaded.

"No," I replied.

"Why not? You're my doctor!"

"It won't help me any."

"You're supposed to be helping me."

"If it won't help me," I said, "then it certainly won't help you."

"But . . . . "

I gave him a precise time and date for his appointment.

He repeated it and hung up.

On my way home that night I stopped in the library for my three volumes. They only had two. Seven and nine. Eight would arrive in a week. I took the two they had home, convinced I would find nothing.

I started with the index of number seven. Nothing.

Then the table of contents. Nothing. No, something. No syrinx, no syringomyelia, but something, a chapter called "Delayed Progressive Myelopathy" by a neurologist from London, Ontario, named Barnett. He worked in the spinal-cord unit of a Canadian VA hospital there.

Delayed Progressive Myelopathy. That was just what Emil had. He had a disorder of his spinal cord (a myelopathy) that had a delayed onset after his original injury and was now progressing.

Delayed Progressive Myelopathy. Now I had a name. Maybe.

I flipped to the article, which described a series of patients. Each of them was just like Emil. Each had developed new symptoms which started just above the level of the old injury and progressed upward. That was what had happened to Emil, and was still happening to him.

What kind of symptoms?

Sensory changes.

Again like Emil.

Pinprick loss. Temperature loss. Pain and temperature. Precisely like Emil. Progressive myelopathy of the center of the cord, of the toothpaste itself. He was not unique, but what did the other patients have? A descriptive title didn't mean anything.

Why did they have a delayed myelopathy?

Why did it progress?

Barnett had discovered a possible explanation for the problem. As one of their first patients got worse and worse, they did a myelogram, an X-ray study of the spinal cord, to see if it would tell them what was wrong. The spinal cord was larger than normal, about twice as thick as it should have been. The neurosurgeon was worried that the enlargement was due to a tumor. He wanted to operate on their patient, open up his back and, if possible, remove any tumor that was there. Barnett could not prove it wasn't a tumor but thought it might be a syrinx—a long tubular fluid-filled cyst.

The surgeon operated. They opened up the patient's back and exposed his spinal cord. It was twice as wide as a normal spinal cord but there was nothing that looked like a tumor. Having nothing else to do, the neurosurgeon put a needle into the distended cord to biopsy some tissue in order to make a diagnosis. All he got was clear, colorless fluid and as it drained out, the cord shrank, returning to normal size in a matter of minutes. That was what would have been expected if it had been a syrinx.

That was the end of the report.

Now I had more than just a name, Delayed Progressive Myelopathy. I knew that Emil Michaels was not unique. Other patients had developed a similar problem years after severe crush injuries of their spinal cords. In all of them it began at the level of the injury and spread upward like an expanding cyst. In all of them it was in the center of the spinal cord like an expanding syrinx, and in one patient it had been shown to be a fluid-filled syrinx.

I knew what was wrong with Emil. He had a delayed, progressive syrinx, a traumatically induced syrinx. How had that process evolved? In order to be certain, I needed to study his spinal cord, but I could make a good guess. The crushed, squeezed toothpaste displaced upward by the original injury eventually degenerated into a meshwork of scar tissue and inflammation, and as it did it formed a cyst that over the years expanded following the path of least resistance, the loose tissue in the center of the cord. That was the same path all expanding syrinxes followed, albeit in the opposite direction in these patients.

I called the Michaels home. Emil answered the phone.

"It's Dr. Klawans," I said.

"What do you want, Doctor?" he asked coldly.

"Undset," I replied.

"Who?"

"Sigrid Undset, the only female Scandinavian novelist to have won the Nobel Prize for literature. Have you read her?"

"No," he responded tentatively.

I hadn't either. "You should. Very few women have won the Nobel Prize for literature."

"I don't like Pearl Buck."

"Who does?" I agreed.

Then after a pause, I began again. I wanted him to meet me at the office the next morning.

"Is there something more you need to learn?"

"No. There is something I may have learned."

"What?"

I told him what I had read. I explained what a syrinx was. If that was what he had, and I thought it was, then we knew that his arms would not become paralyzed.

"How do you prove it, Doc?"

I told him that we needed to do a myelogram.

"Would that really prove it?"

"No. Not a hundred percent. Not enough to publish, but enough to make the diagnosis."

"What would do that?"

"An autopsy," I informed him automatically, without thinking.

The next day I examined him again, as thoroughly as I had the first time, if not more thoroughly. No neurologist had ever been more compulsive. Although the extent of his findings had changed, their nature had not. They still seemed to represent a syrinx. I told him as much and arranged to admit him to the hospital for a myelogram.

I did the myelogram myself. His spinal cord was enlarged, just as the spinal cord of Barnett's patient had been. I was very excited as I showed them to my senior attending neurologist on rounds the next morning.

He wasn't very excited; he'd seen lots of syrinxes in his lifetime.

"Caused by trauma."

Without an autopsy, he reminded me, that was mere conjecture on my part.

Emil was more impressed. "You were right, Doc."

"I guess so," I admitted.

"So what do you do to get me better?"

"Better?"

"Sure! Better. I want to get better. Or at least get no worse."

"I don't know, Emil," I replied. "I just wanted to make the diagnosis. I thought you'd be happy with that and knowing. . . ."

"Doc, you've got to be kidding me."

I wasn't.

"Can't you drain it, or something?"

That was a possibility, but a possibility associated with a risk. Opening the cyst meant operation on the cord in the neck where the cyst was the largest. And a sudden collapse of the cord there could paralyze his arm.

"Why operate there?"

Why indeed? It was where the neurosurgeons always operated on patients with syrinxes. But Emil was different; his syrinx went all the way to L-2. He could be operated on at L-2. If something went wrong there, it was no big deal—he was already paralyzed.

I went off to talk to the neurosurgeons.

No dice.

It was all conjecture on my part. Fantasy. They'd never heard of delayed post-traumatic syringomyelia. No one had. And no one had ever operated on a syrinx at L-2. They looked at the films. They might operate at the neck, but the chances of making the patient worse were one in ten or perhaps two in ten.

Emil opted to go home and feel his syrinx expand. He trusted my logical prognosis rather than the odds of one or two out of ten.

I saw him every two months. He didn't get much worse, but each time he asked the same questions.

"Same diagnosis, Doc?"

"Yes."

"Find anybody willing to cut at L-two yet?"

"No. Have you read Undset yet?"

"I've moved into Proust."

About a year later, I was called to see Emil in the hospital. He had severe renal failure due to his many infections. He was going to die.

"I never found a surgeon," I said.

"I never read any Undset," he admitted.

"Neither have I."

"Doc, this should never happen again. Be sure you do the autopsy and be sure to publish the paper."

I nodded.

Two weeks later Emil Michaels died. We did the autopsy and I studied his spinal cord. He had a scar in his spinal cord where it had been crushed at L-2 and a syrinx which had begun in a small cyst above the scar and had then expanded in the central gray part of the cord from the level of the scar and extended upward the entire length of the spinal cord. I wrote it up as I promised and Emil became my first published paper, the first pathologically studied case of post-traumatic syringomyelia. A few years later, Barnett wrote a book on syringomyelia and put the photographs of Emil's spinal cord in the book. Now everyone knew that such a process existed. The next time I asked a neurosurgeon to operate on a patient like Emil, he was more than willing to do it. And he informed me, as if it were his own idea, he wouldn't operate in the neck but at the level of the old injury.

"Why?" I asked.

"It'll be safer that way. It's what we always do."

I nodded.

"But," he added, "neurologists don't care about such technical issues, do they?"

"Some of us do," I said.

He nodded, unconvinced.

Barrett, by the way, no longer writes about syringomyelia. He is now, and has been for some time, one of the best-known experts on strokes and their prevention and has probably done more than anyone else to prove that aspirin can prevent strokes. I never read one of his papers about strokes without recalling Emil Michaels and the time our paths crossed.

PART TWO

IN SICKNESS AND IN HEALTH

There is only one cardinal rule: One must always listen to the patient.

Oliver Sacks, MD

ALL THE WAY FROM MILWAUKEE

But what of the family?
They know, but are
not talking.

John Stone, MD
Causes

He was my first out-of-town patient. Not just from the suburbs. Or even the far suburbs—the exurbs, or whatever they are called. They are all part of Chicago in my mind. Patients from the suburbs, no matter how far they had to drive to get to my office at the hospital, were not out-of-towners. Albert Coles was an out-of-towner. That could not be debated. He drove all the way from Milwaukee to Chicago to see me. That may not seem that far. Officially, it's only ninety-three miles from the heart of Milwaukee to the center of Chicago. But it's farther than that. Milwaukee is in a different world, with its own industry, its own medical centers, its own baseball teams, its own suburbs, its own life. To Chicagoans, Milwaukee is as remote as Cleveland, Pittsburgh, or Detroit.

Actually, he had not driven that far to see me. He had come all that way in order to be treated with levodopa for his Parkinson's disease. Like so many other patients with Parkinson's disease, he had read all about his miracle drug and I was the closest physician using levodopa. Ninety-three miles is not very far to travel for a miracle. And Albert Coles hadn't actually driven. He could no longer drive himself; his legs were too sluggish. So he arrived with an entourage.

He was in a wheelchair and did not even try to move it himself. One of the two young men with him—sons, I assumed, pushed him into my office. Once there, the two sons stood behind him. A woman in a white uniform sat next to him. A nurse, I supposed. She straightened his tie and brushed off his jacket with her hands. His appearance should not be demeaned by a few flecks of dandruff from the seborrhea common in Parkinson's. Once the dandruff was gone, she clucked with satisfaction.

A very solicitous nurse, I decided.

She smiled at me. I knew that I could now get started. I introduced myself.

She introduced Mr. Coles, patting him on the head as she did.

A solicitous nurse, who had been taking care of him for years.

He was about sixty. She looked to be the same age.

She then introduced his two sons, calling them by their first names and smiling at each of them and finally she introduced herself. She was Mrs. Coles. And she was a registered nurse. And she had dedicated her entire being to taking care of her precious Albert. She did everything for him. She fed him. She shaved him. She dressed him. She bathed him.

She went on and on. If she could have, she would have gone to the toilet for him. As it was, she took him to the bathroom and even held his "little implement" whenever he had to urinate—which was far too often as far as she was concerned. She'd been caring for him in every way for eight years. They'd been married for the last four. She had allowed him to come here. Albert had heard about levodopa on television and in all those magazines. And it had gotten him so excited. Too excited. Such excitement wasn't good at his age. And, well, she didn't believe in miracles. She'd been a nurse far too long to believe in such things. She knew she couldn't help him. Her Albert was too far gone. He hadn't walked by himself in years, but she didn't want to leave any stone unturned. If there was any way to help poor Albert, she wanted to help him.

She'd do anything for him. Once again she started her recitation of everything she did for him and as she did, she smiled at him and patted his hand.

He smiled back.

"Money" she said, "is no problem. Albert's rich. He owns two large breweries. We must do everything we can so that Albert gets better." Then, standing beside him and out of his line of vision, she winked at me once. It was a wink filled with significance, but I wasn't at all certain as to the exact nature of that significance.

Over the next twenty minutes, I obtained the history I needed. Albert Coles was sixty-one years old. He had been born and raised in Milwaukee. He'd lived there all of his life and had been a very successful businessman. He'd enjoyed very good health until he was about forty-seven. At that time, his first wife, the mother of his two sons, was dying of cancer of the breast and he noticed that his right arm felt stiff. So did his right leg. He never went to the doctor. "Such a dear sweet man," the second Mrs. Coles said with a smile and another wink. At the funeral, his right hand shook like a leaf. Nervous exhaustion was his own diagnosis. And everyone else's. The shaking never went away and six months later he was diagnosed as having Parkinson's disease. Within three years, he was having a great difficulty walking, and by the time he was fifty-three, he needed help to take care of himself.

Enter the second Mrs. Coles.

He had trouble zipping his zipper; she'd zip it for him. He had trouble tying his tie, she'd tie it. Windsor or four-in-hand. She'd cut his food. Feed him. Wipe his nose.

Albert tripped once; she put him in a wheelchair. No cane. No walker. No physical therapy for gait instruction. Straight into a wheelchair. She was a nurse; she knew what was best. She knew that falling could be very dangerous. If Albert fell and broke a hip, he might never walk again. So he had to use his wheelchair, even for the shortest walks. After all, didn't most accidents happen at home?

"How long has it been," I asked, "since he walked by himself?"

"We got the wheelchair four years ago," Mrs. Coles replied.

That, I assumed, was supposed to answer my question. Mr. Coles said nothing. She had not given him the chance. She was already going on and on about taking care of his daily needs. "Thank God, he no longer goes to the office. That was such an ordeal. What I had to go through to get him there, day in and day out."

"How long has it been since he's gone to work?"

"Two years," she said. "I finally put my foot down. Enough was enough."

She droned on about how she had sacrificed her life caring for her poor little Albert. I suspected that she had. And I admired her for it. Still, he was my patient. The issue was what I could do for him. Could I get him better? And if so, how much better? Could I get him to walk again? I doubted it. Four years without walking was a very long time. Probably far too long. She had been too caring, too solicitous. The worst thing that patients with Parkinson's disease can do is to stop walking. If their balance becomes impaired, they should walk with assistance or use a cane or a walker. Never a wheelchair unless all other alternatives have failed. Once they give up walking for any period of time, it is very hard for them to learn to walk again.

Not impossible, but very, very difficult. I had had patients who had not walked for three or six months and were started on levodopa and learned to walk again well enough to be independent. But four years? That seemed out of the question.

Mrs. Coles was still talking. I had been lost in my own conjectures. I interrupted her. "It's time for the examination."

"We'll go into the examining room and get undressed."

"No," I said. "I'll take Mr. Coles and I'll examine him."

"But he's used to me. I do everything for him," she protested. "He needs me to do everything for him."

"I'm sure we'll manage," I said, and with that I pushed him down the hall to an examining room.

The examination did not involve much. There were only a few neurologic questions to be answered. Did he have the signs and symptoms of Parkinson's disease? Did he have the signs of anything else that might interfere with his response to treatment? I knew most of the former by watching him and hearing his history. I'd seen his tremor and his mask-like expression. I'd heard all about his stiffness and slowness and lack of balance. I felt his rigidity, checked a few other things. It seemed to me that "her Albert" had Parkinson's disease and nothing more. If only it had been less than four years since he had last walked.

"Three months," he said. His voice was soft, monotonous—Parkinsonian, but I'd heard far worse. He was easy for me to understand.

"What's that?" I asked.

"Three months. It's only been three months since I walked."

It was as if he had been reading my mind.

"How's that?"

There was a glint in his eyes now. It was his turn to wink at me. His voice was stronger with more inflections. "When I went to the office; she left me there all by myself and I walked two miles each day. Around my office. Like a prisoner exercising in a cell."

"But that was two years ago."

"And after that, I'd walk whenever she went out to play bridge. That was twice a week, but she stopped three months ago."

"And no more walking since?"

"Some. A little. I sneak in a few steps here and there but no real walking."

"Why?"

"She likes to take care of me. It keeps her happy. This will be our little secret. I need her. No one could ever take care of me the way she does. Please?" He began to cry.

Fear of being dependent and without help is a powerful force and there was no reason for me to fight it.

"Please," he asked again.

"Of course, Mr. Coles. It's our secret."

I checked a few more reflexes on him. I already knew everything I had to know but I wanted to give him a chance to recover his composure. When he had, I pushed him back into my office, and the five of us had a conference—Albert, his wife, his two sons, and me.

I told them that I thought I could help Mr. Coles. He had Parkinson's disease. There were no contraindications to levodopa and no evidence on examination of any problem other than his parkinsonism. The odds were he would do well.

"But he hasn't walked in four years," his wife interjected. "Doesn't that make it very unlikely that he'll ever walk again? That's what they told us in Milwaukee. Weren't they right? Never again. My poor Albert. I don't want you to give him false hope and then break his heart. That would be a very cruel thing to do, Doctor."

No, I tried to reassure her, there was still a good chance the levodopa would help.

"One out of ten?" she asked.

"Closer to four out of five."

She remained skeptical, but it was agreed that Albert should be admitted to the hospital for a trial of levodopa. It was his best hope. "But we won't expect a miracle," she reminded us all.

Ten days later, Albert Coles was admitted to our hospital. In those days, levodopa was still an experimental drug; its use in Parkinson's disease had not yet been approved by the FDA. Our original protocol had called for us to initiate levodopa therapy in the hospital. It remained like that until levodopa was released for general use, although we knew long before that that levodopa was safe enough to be given without requiring hospitalization. Albert Coles became the seventy-second patient under my care to be given levodopa. I started him the same way I had started all of the others, one quarter of a gram four times a day after food. The levodopa was given after some food because this helped to decrease the tendency of levodopa to cause nausea and vomiting. Decrease, but not eliminate. The next few weeks, I explained to them, would be made up of two progressions. The first would be a slow increase of his daily dosage of levodopa. The rate of this would be dictated by the degree of the side effects it caused.

"I never get sick to my stomach," he told me.

"But you've never taken this," she reminded him. "It works on the vomiting center in your brain. Albert, we have to be very careful."

She was right. Levodopa caused nausea and vomiting by directly stimulating the vomiting center of the brain and because of that we had to go slowly and carefully and wait for the patient to adjust to any one dose before trying to increase the dosage any further. But Albert was also right; patients who never get sick to their stomachs were much more likely to tolerate the levodopa quite well.

"And why is that?" she asked a bit too abrasively.

It was a good question. One I had wondered about before. No one knew the absolute answer, but I had some possible explanations. I gave her one. "The reason they've never been sick to their stomachs before, the reason Albert hasn't, is that their vomiting centers are less sensitive. That's why Albert has never gotten sick to his stomach from other medicine in the past."

"He did once," she objected.

"Why he's only gotten sick to his stomach once before." I amended my explanation and then went on. "The second aspect of our program is daily physical therapy with emphasis on gait training; walking, getting out of a chair by yourself. All of those things you need to do to be totally independent again."

"But he hasn't walked in years," she objected. "Four years."

I did not contradict her.

Nor did Albert.

"It'll never work. It won't help. The very idea. Poor Albert can't walk. He can't get up by himself. He can't stand. I am his legs. His arms. He'll never be independent," she said in a frantic rush. "He can't even hold his own thing when he goes to the bathroom."

"I don't want to be independent," he reassured her. "I just want to be able to walk a little bit. I'll never be able to do so without your help."

She calmed down.

"Physical therapy is part of our program," I told them. "It is part of the protocol. Perhaps it will help; perhaps it won't, but we have no choice."

"I'll go with him," she decided to make sure they didn't push him too hard, make him try too much. "His heart."

"What about his heart?" Neither of them had mentioned anything about heart disease.

"We don't like to talk about that," she said. "I'll only let the therapist do what is good for Albert."

"No," I said. "That's not the way PT works. They and I make the decisions. If Albert has a heart problem, I need to know about it so that I and PT can tailor a program to his needs and ability. We've had experience before in patients with Parkinson's and heart disease. We'll get a cardiology consultation before we start PT."

She scowled.

He nodded. Why, I wondered, had he not told me about his heart disease? Was he afraid that I'd tell him he was too sick for the medicine, for his miracle? That had happened to me before.

That afternoon I learned the answer. He had no heart disease. The cardiologist saw him and gave him a clean bill of health. It was not Albert who had lied to me. He had said nothing. It was his wife who had lied. His wife who was his arms, legs, and mouth. It was not the Parkinson's disease that was going to give me trouble. That was now abundantly clear. Somehow, I was her enemy. I and the levodopa.

At 4:00 P.M. I gave them the good news. We'd start the levodopa after dinner and PT the next morning.

"I think you're going too fast. He's exhausted. That so-called heart specialist was here for two hours. And besides, I'm not sure we believe him. We want another opinion. Who was he? Just a cardiologist you picked?"

"He's the chairman of cardiology here. Last year, he was president of the American Heart Association," I said, knowing that the last was a lie.

"President?" she grumbled. "At least he could have told us who he was."

That night Albert got his first dose of levodopa, the first installment of his salvation.

He got the second with breakfast the next morning. I saw him about an hour after that.

"How are you?" I asked. "Any nausea?"

"We took our pill at about eight-thirty," she said. "And we're pretty good so far, but we may get sick later."

Our pill? I was about to say something but was interrupted by the arrival of someone from transport service. It was time for Albert to go to PT.

"We must go to PT now," she said.

69

"He must go," I reminded her.

"But who will watch out for him?"

"I will," I said. "I will go there personally."

And I did. It was part of my rounds. I had long ago learned that seeing the patients work during physical therapy was one of the best ways to monitor their progress. I got to PT about twenty minutes after Albert did. He was already hard at work. He was walking on the parallel bars, all by himself. There was no therapist holding him up. He was holding himself up. And when he got to the end of the parallel bars, he didn't stand there and wait to be turned with assistance. He turned around by himself, all the time holding on to the bars. His balance was not good enough for him to walk without holding on.

I was pleased. His movements were slow. His steps were shuffling. His posture was stooped. His stride was short. In essence, he was a typical Parkinson patient, but he could walk the bars himself. And that was all I needed. Typically Parkinson patients who were still able to walk and who were started on long-term levodopa treatment responded well. They improved. Their walking improved. So did their balance, their stiffness. That was the miracle he had wanted.

We followed this routine for the six weeks he was in the hospital. I would see them both in his room as I started my daily rounds and then later I would see him performing in PT. Sometimes we talked then; sometimes I just watched him go through his paces. Slowly but steadily, I raised his daily dose of levodopa.

From one gram to one and a half. From one and a half to two.

From two to two and a half. To three. To three and a half.

I waited for five or six days after each increment to make sure his body could tolerate the new level and to observe the effects on his overall function. Each day in the room, Mrs. Coles remained skeptical. Her skepticism was wearying, but it was nothing more than a minor irritation.

"How are you today?" I'd ask.

"He hasn't vomited yet," she'd say.

"Yet? Is he nauseated?"

"Albert never complains, but he didn't finish his second egg. And that means something."

Exactly what that meant was unclear to me. "How did you do yesterday?"

"He is not that much better. We cannot throw away the wheelchair. I still have to dress him completely. I still have to take him to the bathroom and hold his little thing . . . ."

By then, I would turn off her litany and glance through the chart to make sure nothing had gone wrong. The blood tests were all normal. The nurses' notes described nothing unusual. The PT notes gave a picture of progress. Later each morning I personally observed that progress. Albert's strides were longer. He no longer shuffled his feet as he walked. He had a far greater ability to pick up his feet. His turns were far quicker and required fewer steps. He went from a six-step turn with marked shuffling to a four-step turn. Then down to three steps. Two. Then a true pivot, just like non-Parkinson patients do when they turn.

A pivot with only one hand on the bars. Then with no hands. Normal, no evidence of Parkinson's on turning.

The next day he did not even use the bars at all. He started in a chair. He got up by himself, walked across the gym, turned, and walked back across the gym to me. "How am I doing?" he asked with a smile. He knew the answer and he was pleased.

I walked behind him and suddenly pulled backward on his shoulders to test his balance.

He stood in place, as steady as the Rock of Gibraltar. There would be no falls in his immediate future. If they didn't want to throw away the wheelchair, they could certainly put it into storage.

"You're doing terrifically," I said.

He beamed, and as he did, his tongue slowly protruded and his lip twisted to the left ever so slightly. We talked for another couple of minutes. Then I watched him go through the rest of his routine. I watched for fifteen minutes. I saw a total of three abnormal twitches of his lips or tongue. All three were so mild as to be insignificant. They were a sign of an effect of levodopa on the brain, and in a way were a type of toxicity, but virtually all patients get these movements from levodopa and as long as those abnormal movements remained mild, I did nothing. They were not dangerous to the patient and the only way to stop them was to lower the dose of medication and if I did that, the patient usually got worse. If the movements got a lot more severe, I was sometimes forced to do that, but Albert's movements were hardly noticeable.

"Mr. Coles," I asked him, "Why do you let your wife dress you and take you to the bathroom?"

"She loves me. She needs to take care of me. It's her role. And I love her."

He could tell I was not swayed by his explanation.

"And I may need her again to do all those things someday. We

71

don't know if my miracle will last forever."

He was right about that. The longest I had treated anyone with levodopa was about fifteen months. The longest anyone had been treated continuously was about three years. He was right, but did it justify everything she did? That I guess, was a matter of perspective. I just nodded and said nothing.

The next morning on rounds, I started with my usual "How are you this morning?"

"He's terrible. Those horrid mouth movements. That terrible medicine is killing my poor little Albert. It's destroying his brain. His tongue jerks. His lips too. It's grotesque. Hideous. Those movements must hurt horribly. That medicine is poisoning him."

I'd heard enough. His movements were mild, insignificant, more like a minimal tic than the disfiguring spasm she was portraying. "Do they hurt?"

"They must. They look so ugly."

"Do they hurt, Mr. Coles?" I persisted.

"No, but they do bother my wi . . . me," he answered.

I understood. I carefully explained my approach to such movements. Virtually every one of my patients had them. They had to accept them. So did their wives or husbands. As long as they were mild, there was nothing to do.

"Mild!" she burst out. "You call these mild?"

"Yes. They are mild. As long as they don't interfere with his speech or eating, we change nothing." I went on to explain that the only treatment was to reduce the medicine and then we might lose all that we had gained, all the progress.

She then went back to her daily routine. "He is not that much better. We cannot throw away the wheelchair. I still have to dress him completely."

I kept him in the hospital for three more days to make sure that the movements got no worse. They didn't. So I sent him home with an appointment to see me in two weeks.

Two weeks later, they all came to my office: Albert Coles, his wife, his sons.

"He wants to go to work," she complained. "He can't. You tell him, he can't. That he mustn't. That it's not safe. I still have to do everything for him." She started off again.

I stopped her. "He can go to work. If he needs any help, his two sons are there." I turned to them for assent, for support. They said nothing.

"He can return to work," I repeated.

"With those disgusting twists of his face? You have to lower the medicine."

Albert and I walked to the examining room. He looked almost normal. No stiffness, just slightly slow, and the facial movements were still very mild. We talked briefly. He felt great, better than he had in years and he wanted to go back to work. We walked back to my office. There would be no changes in his medicine. And I would see him again in four weeks and he could return to work.

Four weeks later on the morning of his scheduled appointment, I got a phone call from Mr. Coles. He was calling from his office. He'd been back at work for four weeks.

"Too much work?" I suggested.

"No," he replied.

"Is someone sick?"

"No."

I waited for an explanation.

"My sons," he said, his voice choked by emotion, "are too busy to drive me."

"They are?"

"That's what they say."

He asked for an appointment in one week and I gave him one. "You will be able to get driven in then?" I inquired.

He assured me that there would be no difficulty at all. "My sons," he continued, "don't want me here. They think it's their business. That I'm an old man who should have retired years ago, but I'm showing them. This is my business and I'm healthy enough to run it."

One week later, right on time, Mr. and Mrs. Coles arrived at my office. Neither of his sons accompanied them.

Mr. Coles did not look good. Perhaps he was working too hard, I suggested.

He shook his head.

Or perhaps the problems at work, I offered diplomatically, had taken their toll.

"No," he said softly.

"He works too much," she said. "He should stay home. There is no one at work to help him like I do at home. I don't see why he does it. His sons are right. He deserves his retirement. He should stay home with me and let me take care of him. They can take care of the business and I will take care of my Albert. He's worked hard enough for enough years. But he has to go to work every day. And now he

73

has his own chauffeur. He can go where he wants to, whenever he wants to. That's wrong. He must let me take care of him."

I made no comment. Albert was obviously slower and stiffer. I had observed that as he walked into my office. His face was more immobile, less plastic. His voice was softer, slower, more muted. It was obvious that his Parkinsonism was worse. The question was why.

The answer was easy to discover. He was on less levodopa. When I'd seen him five weeks before, he'd been taking three and a half grams per day.

"How much is he taking?" I asked.

"Two and a half grams," she said with a smile.

"Two and a half grams? Why?" I asked.

"Those horrid movements," she said.

"Those mild facial movements?"

"Mild! They were never mild. We could not live with them. We decided to take less medicine."

I was no longer certain who was the doctor, but I gave it another try. "I think he should take more."

"We don't think so," she said.

"We don't?"

"No, we don't!"

I made several other sallies; all of which were easily rebuffed. Finally, I gave them three bottles of levodopa. Mrs. Coles took them and put them in her purse. She was obviously in charge of their medication.

I told them to come back in six weeks.

About ten minutes later as I was seeing another patient, someone knocked on the door of my office. I opened the door. It was a man in his sixties whom I did not recognize.

"I am Albert Coles' driver, and his best friend. We went to high school together," he said.

"Is anything wrong?"

"Al left his hat."

I looked on my desk. His hat was there. I picked it up and gave it to his old friend.

"He also says he needs another bottle of medication, to be on the safe side."

"He has enough."

"In case it snows and he can't get back."

Snows? It was August. "But . . . ."

"To be on the safe side, to be sure," he interrupted me.

I understood. "You better take two bottles," I said. "It's experimental. He can't get it anywhere else." I gave him two bottles.

"Albert says he forgot how much you wanted him to take each day."

"Three grams a day," I said.

"Three grams a day," he repeated.

"Yes."

That was the way the next three visits went. The Coles came in. I talked to them. I examined him. He was doing well, as well as he had on his first return visit. No slowness, no stiffness. His balance was good. And he had an occasional, mild, insignificant facial grimace. She told me how much medicine he was on. Two and a half grams, then two, then one and a half. She'd complain that he shouldn't be so independent. The sons could run the business. He should stay at home. She could take care of him. As it was, he was going to work seven days a week. Seven days! Wasn't that too much? He was a sick man. And then she'd go into a tirade about those horrid movements.

After I'd listen as long as I could, I'd give her the levodopa and watch her lock it into her purse.

Then ten minutes later there would be a knock on my door. It would be Al's best friend.

Al had forgotten something. A hat. A briefcase. Something. Whatever it was was on my desk.

"Al wonders if the three grams a day is enough?"

"It is."

"And he'd like some more medicine."

"To be on the safe side," I'd add as I gave him the medication.

Mrs. Coles was obviously giving him one and a half grams a day at home, and he was giving himself the other one and a half grams. That was why he went to work seven days a week; not to work, but to take his medicine. He was on three grams a day and doing very well, with occasional mild, abnormal facial movements. But, overall, "we" were doing quite well.

On the last of these three visits, there was a slight variation. Mrs. Coles added a new complaint. She was afraid that Mr. Coles was developing psychosis from his levodopa.

"Psychosis?" I inquired. He seemed very much in touch with reality to me.

"His personality is changing. He doesn't trust me the way he used to. He is much too independent. He wants to go to the bathroom himself. He even tries to dress himself. He gets angry when I remind him that he can't do those things. Angry at me! After all I have done for him. All of the sacrifices I have made for him."

It was the same old record with just a minor twist. The levodopa was affecting Albert's mind and driving him crazy. Levodopa can cause a psychosis, but that kind of psychosis is associated with hallucinations and confusion. Albert was not having hallucinations. He was not confused.

"We are going crazy from that poison," she concluded.

"Albert is not psychotic." I said. "And levodopa is not a poison. I will see you in two months."

Two months later Albert Coles called me on the morning of his appointment. His friend had been fired or bought off by his family or both. he wasn't certain of the details. All he knew was that someone had discovered his supply of medicine at his office and taken it. This had happened the day before. Then this morning, his friend did not come by to pick him up and drive him to work and then to see me. They had planned to ask me for some more "extra" medication.

"That won't be a problem," I reassured him.

He was pleased.

"But how are you going to get here and get it?"

He wasn't sure. He might just call a limousine service or call another old friend, but he would get here. He might be late, but he'd get to my office. He needed the levodopa. "How late are you there?" he asked.

"Five-thirty, six," I told him.

"I'll get there."

"I'll wait for you."

"You won't have to," he assured me and hung up.

That afternoon I was quite busy. I didn't even think about Albeit Coles until a little after five, as I started to see my last patient. It was then that I realized that he had not yet gotten to my office.

I bade my last patient goodbye at a little before five-thirty. There was still no sign of Albert Coles. I'd wait. I had work to do and several phone calls to return to other patients.

Six o'clock and still no Albert Coles.

Six-fifteen.

Six-thirty. I had returned all the calls, dictated all the notes and letters that I had to dictate, answered all my mail. I'd wait another fifteen minutes, I decided.

At six forty-five, I called him at his office. There was no answer. I called his home. Again, there was no answer. They had to be on the way, I decided.

Seven.

Seven-fifteen. I called again, both numbers, and again got no reply.

At seven-thirty, I locked up and went home. I'd call him at the office the next day. We could always send him the medicine by UPS and I could see him in a week or two.

At about two the next morning, my phone rang.

"Dr. Klawans," the male voice said. It was not a voice I recognized.

"Yes," I yawned, looking at the clock and wondering what kind of an emergency had prompted this call.

"This is William Coles, Albert's older son. I've seen you at your office a couple of times."

"What's wrong?" I asked.

"It's Dad. He's gone crazy."

"Crazy?" I repeated. Perhaps Mrs. Coles had been right. Perhaps the levodopa had been affecting Albert's mental processes and he had been clever enough to hide it from me.

"Yes. He's psychotic. He's out of his mind. We have to admit him to a psychiatric unit. He's out of control. It's the levodopa. It's made him crazy."

"Crazy?" I repeated once again. "In what way?"

William Coles repeated his vague generalizations. His father was crazy. Psychotic, out of control. He had to be admitted and taken off levodopa. That poison had driven him insane.

Poison? It was the same word Mrs. Coles had used to describe levodopa. Very few people called medications poisons.

"He's out of control. He can never take that poison again."

"Perhaps," I said.

"He's crazy," William Coles repeated.

"In what way?" I insisted. "Describe it to me."

"He's violent."

"Violent?"

"Yes. He's completely out of his mind."

"In what way was he violent?"

"He struck Mrs. Coles."

"Struck her?"

"Yes. Tonight. She was taking him to the bathroom and for no

77

reason at all he hit her."

Hit her one for me, Al baby, I thought.

"He's dangerous. You must do something."

"I'll tell you what. You bring him in to see me at eight o'clock this morning and I'll do whatever I can to help him. We may put him in this hospital here and I'll make sure we straighten everything out. I'm sure I can get him over this."

They never brought him in to see me that next morning. Or ever again. I never saw him again. When I called the next day, I was told that he had a new doctor. I was no longer his physician.

I'd been fired. "Who is his doctor?" I inquired, trying to be as polite as I could under the circumstances.

"Someone who understands his needs better," the voice responded. It was William Coles' voice.

"Give me the doctor's name so I can send him the medicine."

"What medicine?"

"The levodopa."

"The doctor won't need your levodopa."

"But Albert can't get levodopa from any doctor in Milwaukee," I protested.

"That poison is not what he needs. He needs our love and care and protection." And with that the younger Coles hung up.

I tried calling several more times, but got nowhere and I let it drop at that. What else could I do? I had other problems to keep me busy; patients whose families wanted them to be healthy. In a few weeks, Albert Coles was all but forgotten, except for the punch line. That became an anecdote I told many times: Hit her one for me, Al baby. Hit her one for me.

Five years later I learned the real punch line, by accident. I had been referred another patient from Milwaukee. By then that no longer seemed exotic to me. I called the referring physician to discuss the options since the patient's Parkinson's disease was complicated by several other medical conditions. After we talked for a few minutes and seemed to have reached agreement on a course of action, the doctor changed the subject.

"I hope this patient does better than the last patient I sent to you."

"Who was that?" I inquired sheepishly.

"Albert Coles."

"How is he?"

"He's been dead for two years."

"Dead?"

"Yes."

"For two years? How? Why?"

"Pneumonia. His Parkinson's got the best of him."

"Oh, I see."

"It was too bad that the levodopa made him so violent. We stopped it. We were all afraid to start it again."

"But it wasn't the—" I started to protest.

"I know you like levodopa, but it made him crazy. Psychotic. And poor Mrs. Coles, that saint of a woman. She cared for him twenty-four hours a day. She watched him like a hawk. But despite all of her efforts, the disease was too severe. And we could not use levodopa. We couldn't put that dear woman through that again. And besides it never helped him that much. It caused such severe facial movements and then such destructive behavior. To him, it was a poison."

THE COLLECTOR

When I am in my painting, I'm not aware of what I'm doing . . . because the painting has a life of its own.

Jackson Pollock

I'm in my element when I'm a little bit out of this world: Then I'm in the real world—I'm on the beam. Because when I'm falling, I'm doing all right; when I'm slipping, I say, hey, this is interesting! It's when I'm standing upright that bothers me: I'm not doing so good; I'm stiff.

Willem De Kooning

We became friends because we shared a passion. We both love and collect contemporary art and have discovered an unlikely parallel in our tastes: French abstract art since the Second World War and nonabstract American art of the same era. But our collections could not be more dissimilar. Walter Harley and his wife owned major works by such French luminaries as Dubuffet, Braque, Arman, while my wife and I had etchings and lithographs by Atlan, Singer, and Dubuffet. Their American works were by Lichtenstein, Johns, Stella, Diebenkorn—a coast-to-coast selection of the who's who of modern American art, while we collected Chicago artists, Ed Paschke, Roger Brown, Vera Klement, William Conger. We had met because he had a neurologic problem and a mutual friend, the director of one of Chicago's best-known art galleries had suggested that I might be able to help him. And so he became my patient.

He had one of those neurologic problems just beginning to "come out of the closet." Not that what he had was a new disease. Far from it, it is one of the "older" neurologic disorders, the existence of which goes back at least as far as the great sixteenth-century Dutch genre painter, Pieter Bruegel the elder. Bruegel often filled his scenes of sixteenth-century Dutch village life with a staggering variety of local characters, including especially the injured, the deformed, the diseased, and the disabled. One of these portrait-caricatures illustrated an old man with the neurologic disorder I diagnosed in Walter Harley. Bruegel did that some four hundred years before any physician bothered to differentiate this disorder from all the other maladies of mankind and give it the status of a specific disease, one we now call Meige's syndrome, after the medical observer Henri Meige, not Bruegel's disease. Bruegel had simply observed all the manifestations, abstracted them, and reproduced them in a picture.

What Meige described was a form of dystonia, a term used medically today to classify a group of abnormal movements that share the same characteristics—slow, spontaneous, abnormal movements that tend to form fixed postures. Not sudden brief jerks or rhythmic tremors, but movements that hold a posture. In Meige's syndrome these dystonic movements, usually beginning in middle adult life, affect the muscles around the eye, the mouth, and the jaw, less often the tongue. The patients all tend to have similar problems, among them spontaneous, prolonged, uncontrollable eye closure, now called blepharospasm, associated with a peculiar appearance due to distortions of the lips and lower face and displacement of the jaw to one side or the other, resulting in chewing problems.

The picture that illustrated Meige's original article, a photograph of my patient, and the painting done by Bruegel all show the same features: deeply furrowed eyebrows and wrinkled nose with eyes tightly clamped shut, a distorted mouth, and a jaw jutting to one side. The disease has not changed in four hundred years, probably much longer. It is unlikely, after all, that Bruegel painted the first such patient, no more likely than the notion that Meige described the first patient, or that he discovered a new disease.

This disease may not have changed, but there's been an increasing recognition on the part of both physicians and patients, especially the latter, that this is a "real" disease. The abnormal dystonic movements that typify Meige's are not entirely random. They do not just come and go in a hit-or-miss fashion. They do that, of course, but far too often they are brought about by activity. *Action-induced* is the term neurologists like to append to the movements: action-induced dystonia. The patient tries to chew and his jaw juts to one side, chewing becomes difficult, food cannot be retained in the mouth.

Walter Harely's action dystonia mostly involved his eyes. Whenever he most needed to keep them open, they started to close. Suddenly, spontaneously, uncontrollably. At first they only closed occasionally and briefly, more an aggravation than a disability. But the problem progressed. The eye closures occurred more and more frequently, and each single closure seemed to be more persistent. They lasted longer; not just a second or two, but, five, ten, fifteen seconds—even longer. The movements were also more forceful and disruptive. At first they tended to occur while he was watching TV or a movie and trying to concentrate on what he was watching. Then his eyes would close tightly while reading a book. He reached the point that his eyes would clamp shut whenever he tried to drive his car. At first these movements were brief and infrequent. But they too progressed so that whenever he tried to drive, his eyes shut, abruptly, without warning, and stayed shut for five, ten, fifteen seconds.

I remember that first appointment. I'd seen him in the waiting room trying to read a book. All at once his eyes had clamped shut like some primitive animal trap. At first, his forehead became deeply furrowed and his eyebrows all but touched his eyelashes. As he tried to open his eyes, his forehead became smooth, his eyebrows lifted, then his eyes finally opened. It all took about a dozen seconds. He looked around the room. As he did, his jaw protruded ever so slightly.

"Meige's," I said to myself.

Ten minutes later he was sitting in my office across the desk from me, outlining his problems. I listened politely and then examined him perhaps a bit too perfunctorily. After all, observing the movements and then listening to his complaints were all that was really necessary in order to make the diagnosis.

Once I had finished examining him and we had returned from the examining room to my office, I told him what he had: Meige's syndrome. A neurologic disease.

"So it's not psychiatric?" he asked.

"No," I assured him.

I tried to explain exactly what dystonias are, since Meige's is a form of dystonia. Explaining dystonia is not a simple task because we know so little about it. We believe that all dystonias are a result of disease of the brain, or the so-called extrapyramidal system of the brain, a very old, primitive motor system that controls postures. For some reason, this system goes haywire and groups of muscles start forming new postures. If the neck turns we call it torticollis; if the eyes close, blepharospasm or Meige's.

He had Meige's.

"Can you help me?" he asked me..

I thought I could. I outlined a course of medications we would try.

He had one more question. "Can I drive my car?"

"Not between here and my house," I told him.

He has now been my patient for nine years and for the last six we've also been friends. The medications I prescribed have given him about eighty percent relief. He blinks more frequently than normal while driving, but the blinks are now brief like normal blinks and he never has any periods of sustained eye closure as long as he doesn't drive for more than half an hour.

It had taken about nine months to find the right combination of medications and then he'd come in for routine follow-up visits once every three or four months. Since he was doing well and wanted no further changes in his medication, the medical aspects of these visits required only a couple of minutes. The rest of the time we talked about other subjects, which quickly narrowed down to the single, but to us inexhaustible, subject of contemporary art.

Then one afternoon he asked, "Do you know De Kooning?"

What a question! He's one of the three or four best known of all American artists and one of the most expensive. He and Jackson Pollock were the two fathers of American abstract expressionism. Of course I knew De Kooning. Who didn't?

That was not what he had meant. He wondered if I knew De Kooning personally.

No. Was there any reason, in particular, why I should?

Of course. I was a neurologist and De Kooning had a neurologic disease. Perhaps he had come to see me. Or vice versa.

I shook my head. "What disease?"

"Alzheimer's."

"My God! That's too bad. I guess there will be no more De Koonings."

"That's where you're wrong. He's still painting as well as ever."

"That's preposterous unless he's in the very, very early stages."

"No, his disease is far advanced, from what I've heard," Walter informed me.

"And he's still painting?"

"Yes."

"Well, either the diagnosis is wrong or there is something rotten in the studio of De Kooning."

"Or perhaps you don't understand the brain and abstract expressionism as well as you think you do."

"I . . . ."

"Come to dinner on Friday with your wife and we'll discuss this

84

in more detail," he said, concluding his visit.

At the dinner table, I sat opposite a large late Dubuffet oil, its small white spaces surrounded by thick black lines and a bright, colored, puppetlike figure similarly encased. I had a similar piece, but mine was a lithograph. My wife sat opposite a De Kooning, a big, bright work filled with bold streaks of color and featuring the figure of a large-breasted woman.

He saw that I could not take my eyes off the De Kooning. "Woman, four," he said.

Woman IV proclaimed both the historical significance and monetary worth of the piece. It had been one of the pivotal series of paintings done in the early fifties when De Kooning introduced figures into abstract expressionism.

Over dinner our conversation quite naturally turned to the subject of De Kooning and his supposed Alzheimer's disease. Walt brought it up. "De Kooning does have Alzheimer's. There is no question about the diagnosis."

I did not know where to start. We are never one hundred percent certain of the diagnosis of Alzheimer's until the patient dies and we can examine the brain itself. Short of that Alzheimer's is a diagnosis of exclusion. The patient has dementia. Alzheimer's is one of those diseases that causes dementia. Its official name today is senile dementia of the Alzheimer's type. SDAT. The name tells all. The patient clinically has a senile dementia, a dementia beginning in mid- or late adult life. And to the clinical observer, the dementia looks and acts like many other dementias. It is the specific changes that can be seen when the brain tissue is examined microscopically that show which type of senile dementia caused the problem.

We order tests on patients not to prove they have SDAT, but to prove whether or not they have other, treatable form of dementia: vitamin deficiency, pernicious anemia, thyroid disease, syphilis, brain tumors, and so on. Once these have been ruled out and the brain scan shows only a loss of brain tissue (brain atrophy), the most likely diagnosis is SDAT. Most likely; not proved. There is a difference. The first step, of course, is to prove that the patient truly has dementia. To neurologists, dementia has a rather specific meaning. To us, dementia means a diffuse loss of all intellectual functions, memory, judgment, learning, whatever the brain does. And the loss is a progressive one. The loss is diffuse and involves most aspects of intellectual function because the disease process is diffuse. The entire brain is involved.

I started to explain all of this to my host. I told him that the diagnosis could only be proved after the death of the patient.

He smiled, unimpressed. "His doctors have told him and his family that he has SDAT."

"How bad is his dementia?" I asked.

Harley told me about the competency hearing that had been held in a Long Island courtroom more than a year before. According to the testimony, De Kooning could read but he could not recall what he read or understand it. He could still do some things. If he was given a toothbrush, he brushed his teeth; a razor, he shaved. The court declared him incompetent.

Courts do not do that without strong evidence. Obviously De Kooning was too incapacitated to manage his own affairs and yet I, and the buying public, were being asked to believe that he was still capable of painting creatively. I didn't.

"At that same hearing, his daughter testified that he still painted every day of the week. And that he painted masterfully. She also testified that he was not competent to manage anything."

"And was, of course, named conservator."

"Co-conservator."

"And she is his heir."

"Yes."

"Not exactly an unbiased witness," I said.

"Perhaps not."

"Each of those new De Koonings would be worth several hundred thousand dollars to her."

"Yes," he conceded. "Perhaps even more."

"There is a fancy neurologic term for the isolated preservation of a complex intellectual, creative activity in a patient with dementia," I said, and waited.

"And what is that?"

"BS. Or as Jack Warner put it, in two short words: Im possible."

"Are you certain of that?"

I was and I tried to explain why once again. SDAT is a diffuse process. Everything goes. It is not like a single stroke in which only one small part of the brain is injured. The whole brain is losing cells. Those cells are dying prematurely.

"Not just the left side?" he asked.

I explained that this was a misconception of pop psychology. There is no neurologic evidence that creativity is localized in either side of the brain exclusively. Not at all. If it were, then there would have been cases that proved it. We, as neurologists, know that speech—speech—not intellectual function—is located on the left side of the brain and in specific parts of the left side because patients with strokes to those areas can lose speech and speech only. And we know that there is a specific area again on the left for mathematical skills because there have been patients with the sudden loss of the ability to carry out calculations who were otherwise absolutely normal and who had had strokes in that area. "Yet," I continued, "there has never been a patient who has lost his creativity and nothing else. It is not a localized function."

"But," he countered, "abstract expressionism is not an intellectual function."

"It isn't?"

"You say that SDAT is a diffuse disease of all realms of intellect."

I nodded.

"And therefore De Kooning cannot paint."

"True."

"And I tell you that to him, painting is not an intellectual function."

"That can't be true."

He quoted Jackson Pollock to me and then such art critics as Clement Greenberg and Harold Rosenberg. It may have been good art criticism, but it was bad neurology. Perhaps Rosenberg was right. Abstract expressionism was an emotional process, an existentialist act in which the artist struggles with his materials for self-creativity, self-awareness, self-definition. That each canvas produced a moment of truth. Perhaps that was all true, but even if it were, De Kooning was no longer competent to recognize that truth.

"But it's not intellectual, it's emotional. He paints with emotion."

"Remember what André Breton said," he continued, invoking the founder of the surrealist movement. "Let me remind you he felt that creativity depended upon what he called 'psychic automatism.'" Creativity did not depend on the exercise of control by reason or intellect but upon the release of creative energies by the unconscious.

"I know. That was the credo of the Surrealist Manifesto. It had no neurologic basis then or now."

"But that's how De Kooning paints—psychic automatism."

"Let me tell you a story. I have an uncle. He's really not my uncle

87

but I call him uncle. He and his wife were our neighbors, my parents' best friends. He has SDAT. Severe SDAT. He's been in a nursing home for six years. Maybe longer. He recognizes no one, not even his son. He developed some signs of Parkinson's and I was asked to see him. I prescribed some medication. Two days later, his son went to visit him. He was seated in a chair in the hallway. As soon as his son got off the elevator, my uncle looked at his son and said 'Look who's here. My best friend.' The son was amazed. The voice had such warmth in it. Such emotion. He thought I was a miracle worker. His father had not recognized him in two years.

"Then the elevator door opened and someone else got out.

"'Look who's here,' the old man said with equal glee, 'my best friend.' That's psychic automatism. Hardly a creative process. Does De Kooning recognize his family?"

"He doesn't even know that his wife is dead."

"I rest my case. He can't still be painting."

"He brushes his teeth."

"So can a three-year-old, but that three-year-old cannot look at a blank canvas and recognize a moment of truth."

We talked about De Kooning only once more, about three months later in my office. Walter started by reading me something Conrad Fried, De Kooning's brother-in-law, had said. According to Fried, in order to understand what was going on you had to realize that De Kooning had been compulsively involved with painting all his life. "It's like he's on automatic pilot, and it doesn't make any difference whether he knows what he's doing or not. He always thought that if you knew what you were doing, you were going in the wrong direction, because then it's just craft. After you've driven a car for thousands of miles, you don't have to think about how to brake or steer. He knows automatically what to do and how to do it."

But I too, had done my homework. There was someone I could quote, abstract-expressionist Richard Pousette-Dart. Pousette-Dart believed that true art was the "complete realization of one's being, a matter of exquisite focus, awareness, consciousness." He didn't believe that the part of the brain responsible for painting is separate. Neither did I.

Walter had read the same statement. "I returned the De Kooning I had just bought. It cost over six hundred thousand dollars."

"Because of what I said? Did I convince you he couldn't really still be painting creatively?" The triumph of neurology over emotionality.

"Not entirely." There were two other factors. It was clear that whatever creative process was going on within that studio filled with assistants and nurses but where no outsiders were allowed in to see exactly who was doing what was not to be trusted. But the other factor had been more significant.

"What was that?" I asked.

"The court had taken away De Kooning's driver's license."

9

IMPRESSING MRS. DASTUR

My first realization of the horror associated with this word came in the year 1934. At a large medical center, I saw a woman who came for diagnosis of a nodular skin eruption. She had lived for a number of years in the tropics and had been told that she had "leprosy." An exhaustive examination, however, revealed a cancer with multiple metastases to the skin. When this condition was explained to the patient her response was unforgettable: "Thank God it's nothing but cancer!"

Frederick C. Landrum, MD

Whenever a patient calls the office to make an appointment to see me for a neurologic evaluation, the receptionists fill out a sheet full of required information. Most of this is what they and our business office call demographics, the sort of information that is needed for billing purposes. The last two blanks are the only two I'm interested in and I always read them before I ever greet the patient. First, why has the patient come to see me? In other words, what do they think is wrong with them? And the second, why me? How were they referred here?

Mrs. Dastur had been asked the same set of questions and I had read her answers before I ever set eyes upon her. She had come to see me because her right hand had lost its feeling. The complaint automatically triggered a set of possible diagnoses in my mind. I assumed that her complaint was both accurate and complete. To me, that meant that her hand had lost feeling but that the sensory loss was limited to the right hand and was not accompanied by weakness in that hand. These were, of course, assumptions on my part, assumptions that would have to be confirmed or refuted when I took her history and examined her in detail. But my mental gymnastics set to work on her chief complaint, a pure sensory loss limited to one hand. For anatomic reasons, that complaint could not be due to disease deep within the brain itself. The sensory tracts as they wind their various ways through the brain to reach the cerebral cortex are such small, tight bundles that it's impossible to destroy feeling from one hand without also altering sensation from the arm and leg on the same side. It's only on the surface of the brain, the cortex, that the sensory messages from the various parts of the body spread out so that each area of the body has its own specific location. The sensory area of the brain lies just behind the motor area and can be mapped out into a homunculus, a manlike creature whose shape is determined by the order and relative sizes of the individual sensory areas. The mouth of the homunculus is large, with protruding lips. The hand is equally out of proportion to the small shoulders and chest. The body is standing on its head, the enormous thumb resting on the tips of the lips and the small legs and feet reaching up to the top of the brain.

This little man was first discovered in the 1870s. This region of the cortex is the one place in the brain where the sensory fibers are spread out enough to allow a disease to injure just a part of the sensory system, but there are limitations as to what can happen. If the hand loses all of its feeling, if the thumb is "dead," then there is always some change in the lips. And two other anatomic facts are equally significant. The sensory area and its neighboring motor strip are not segregated; they are integrated. Not fully, but enough so that a marked loss of one function is always associated by some involvement of the other. Paralysis with some numbness or a dead hand with some mild weakness. She had only complained of a hand that had lost feeling, not strength, not agility, not cunning.

But perhaps I was reading too much into her complaint. Or too little. The other rule is that the cortex does not house all sensations. Pain is not felt in the cortex. Touch, yes. Position sense, where a part of the body is in space, sensory localization, precisely where an object is touching the body, the ability to judge the size, shape, or weight of an object held in the hand, the ability to tell how many objects are touching the skin and how close they are to each other; all of these, which require some sort of "judgment," are found in the sensory cortex. But not pain; that is found deep in the brain, in the thalamus. The thalamus is a relay station which receives the various sensory tracts and relays them to the cortex, but not pain. That stops in the thalamus. A patient without a sensory cortex still feels pain. That patient will not feel a touch, not know where his hand is in space, but pain is still pain and it is still felt, it still enters consciousness.

92

And Mrs. Dastur? Her hand had lost all feeling. That, to me, meant she had lost the ability to transmit pain to the thalamus. Patients who can feel pain but not touch, complain that their hand is numb, not that it has lost all of its feeling. Or was I overreading a spontaneous remark to my receptionist? It didn't matter. This was in part just an exercise for my brain. A workout before the real game. Batting practice.

The brain was probably out. That left the nerves themselves coming up from the hand to go into the spinal cord and the spinal cord where the various sensory pathways began to separate from one another. The list of diagnostic possibilities was long. I spent several minutes going over that list. I hoped my assumptions had been valid; it was an interesting list of diagnoses that I had put together. It would be fun figuring out exactly which one fit her like a glove.

The day of the appointment came and with it the moment of truth. Would my list have to be cast aside and a new one created or not? There were two key questions to be asked, two assumptions to be tested. Were her right leg and the right side of her face spared? Was there any weakness? Batting practice was over. The game had begun.

Mrs. Dastur told me that she was from India. Southern India. I wasn't sure what difference it made whether she was from northern or southern India, and I didn't ask. This was, I assumed, all background. She was fifty-seven. She was a mathematician. She had studied in England, at Cambridge, and then gone back to teach at a university in India, in southern India. She now taught in Chicago and had for the last eight years. She had not been back to India in eleven years, but that was not too long, was it?

"Too long for what?" I asked.

"You know."

I did?

She went on. Her right hand was becoming senseless. It had lost its feeling.

"Is it . . . ," I started.

"It, of course, is not weak," she went on, ignoring my attempt to even ask a question. I'd been right. No weakness.

"And obviously, my right leg is normal."

Right again, but why obviously?

"And miraculously, my face is . . . still my face."

"Of course," I said.

"But that's rare," she contradicted me.

"Not at all." I then explained the anatomy of the homunculus and why sparing her face was not rare; it just meant that her brain was not the site of her disease. All very erudite and self-satisfied, and why not? She'd given a one-sentence reply to a routine question from a receptionist. And I had constructed a differential diagnosis and an entire plan for evaluation based on that reply and a few assumptions. And I'd been right.

"But," she protested, "my brain is normal. There is nothing wrong with my brain. I know that."

I too knew that her brain was normal. So I listed the differential diagnoses of what she could have, from amyloidosis, a rare condition of the nerves themselves, to xanthomatosis, an even rarer cause of disease of the nerves. I left out nothing that I'd ever seen.

"I have none of those things," she said.

If she already knew what she had, then why did she have to come to see me, I wondered.

"I'm from southern India."

Back to southern India again. What difference did that make?

"I have . . . ." She stopped. Before my eyes, this proud, erect, well-educated professor of mathematics, crumbled. She slumped down into the chair, looking more like a beggar on the streets of Calcutta holding out a deformed hand for a few rupees. A hand mangled and deformed by—

"Leprosy." I blurted out without even thinking.

"I am as good as dead. Worse," she replied, having accepted my guess as her final diagnosis.

Leprosy!

So that's why southern India was important. Leprosy is more common there than it is in northern India. And it's still a common disease. There were, I knew, fifteen or twenty million lepers in the world. That made it a very common disease. One hell of a lot more common than amyloidosis or xanthomatosis and everything else I'd put on my list. A list without leprosy on it. Leprosy may well be a common disease in the world, but not in my office.

I understood all of her answers now. She was waiting for her face to become swollen, thickened, deformed, as it did so often. To become less human, more animal-like, elephantine. Thickened, expressionless, frozen, grotesque.

Leprosy.

She sat there defeated, shaking. She lifted her right hand toward me to show off the marks of her disease. Of her leprosy. So much for my differential diagnosis and my extended work-up.

She had leprosy and she knew it and she'd come to me because I was not affiliated with her university. She wanted a private confirmation of her fate. A confirmation she would pay for in cash. It was not something she was willing to acknowledge yet.

I started to tell her about the new treatments, the modern . . . .

"Have you seen many lepers?"

"No."

"I have." She was struggling to regain her composure. Her hand was still extended toward me, no longer begging for alms, but demanding attention, concern. She had a biblical disease, a disease that demanded respect and prayers as much as it caused fear and disgust.

I looked down at her hand. It looked like a normal hand, aside from three or four scars, all fairly new and broad.

"Burns?" I asked.

She nodded.

"Burns you never felt?"

Another nod.

I reached out and held her hand and as I did I was able to get her to tell me her story. For the last year now she had been unable to feel pain with her right hand. She had first realized that when she had cut her finger. Since then, she'd cut herself several times and burned herself half a dozen times.

Her left hand? I inquired.

Normal.

Her strength?

Normal.

Agility?

Fine.

Right foot? Face? Right arm? Right leg?

All uninvolved.

Touch? Could she feel things that just touched her right hand?

Yes.

Normally?

She wasn't certain.

I told her to close her eyes and with a key I drew a number four on her palm. "What number was that?" I asked.

"A four."

I drew a six.

"Six or nine, dependent."

An eight.

"Eight."

I put a nickel in her hand and closed her hand.

"What was that?"

"A nickel."

A key.

"A key."

A safety pin.

Correctly identified once more.

With her eyes still closed, I grasped her thumb and told her to tell me which way I was moving her thumb. I moved her thumb five degrees upward.

"Up," she said.

Then two degrees down.

"Down."

"You can't feel pain," I told her.

That she already knew.

"But you can feel everything else."

That she also knew. Pain is carried in the nerves by small, thin fibers and these are more easily destroyed in leprosy than the thicker fibers that carry touch and position, but not exclusively so. To lose all pain sensation and yet have all else spared would be rare in leprosy. Very rare. I told her that.

She was unimpressed. She'd seen leprosy. Had I? She was from southern India. She knew.

And in leprosy, the nerves were thickened. I felt her hand, behind her elbows. Her neck. Her nerves were not. I told her as much.

So what? She had leprosy. Her life was finished.

Nothing I said could impress her. She knew she had leprosy. She was cursed for life. Treatment was irrelevant. The diagnosis was the curse. The stigma.

Didn't I know the Bible?

That I did know. Well enough to know that biblical leprosy was not the leprosy Mrs. Dastur "knew" she had. There was no leprosy in biblical Israel, despite what the New Testament claimed. The leprosy of the Bible was not a specific disease. It was not a medical problem, it was a religious issue.

"Leviticus," She said.

"That was not leprosy."

She looked at me incredulously. Not only did I not know leprosy, I was a heretic.

96

"In Leviticus, leprosy is described as white. The skin in leprosy is never white. You are from southern India. You know leprosy. Did you ever see white leprosy?" I asked.

She hadn't.

"And in Leviticus, leprosy involves the scalp. In southern India, have you ever seen leprosy of the scalp?"

She hadn't.

I had once more convinced myself that the leprosy of Leviticus was not leprosy at all, but a collection of nonspecific skin diseases. Mrs. Dastur, however, remained unimpressed.

I pressed on. Leviticus had described leprosy on the wall of a house that made that house ritually impure in the same way that leprosy of the skin made a priest impure.

Of course, she had never seen leprosy of the wall of a house. Nor had anyone in southern India, or anywhere else.

"Therefore, the skin affliction in the Bible was not leprosy," I told her.

"But it is called leprosy in my Bible."

"In an English translation of a Greek translation of the Hebrew. The word *leprosy* does not appear in the Hebrew Bible. God never used that word. Not once. Not in Leviticus, or Deuteronomy. The Hebrew word is *sara'at*."

I was no longer a heretic.

"What was this *sara'at* if not leprosy?"

"That's a very good question. Leviticus is not a medical textbook. It never really gives us a full description of *sara'at*. It's a priestly manual. It tells us how a priest should decide if something or someone has *sara'at* or not, but whatever it is, it affects humans, clothes, and houses. And it does not kill people, it's not incurable. It just makes them 'unclean' or impure. Unable to perform certain rituals."

"And so unclean that they had to live outside of the camp."

She, too, knew her Leviticus.

"But why does my Bible call it leprosy?"

I tried to explain the confusion to her. How a rather diffuse concept of ritual uncleanliness that applied equally to a number of human skin disorders, garments, and houses, came to be attached to a single, specific disease that still existed and whose victims still suffered from the same biblical taint, from the admonition that they had to live outside the camp.

Leprosy was not a national curse. It was not bubonic plague. Or smallpox, measles, typhus, cholera, typhoid. These diseases could threaten an entire tribe. A whole nation. A people. Leprosy could not do that. Its curse is personal, not national.

"The word," she said.

"The Hebrew Bible was first translated into Greek for the library at Alexandria under Ptolemy IV, in the third century before Christ, by seventy scholars, scholars who knew Hebrew, the Bible, and Greek. That's how the word *septuagint* originated. Septuagint. Seventy. They had a lot of words they had to wrestle with. *Sara'at* was one of them. They picked the word *lepra*. Not leprosy, lepra."

"Leprosy already existed then and Greek physicians had a word for it. That word was not *lepra,* it was *elephas* or elephantiasis: because of the elephantine appearance of the face deformed by the thick nodules characteristic of the disease. *Elephas,* not *lepra.* That word was used by them all. Celsius, Galen, even Pliny the Elder."

"*Elephas,*" I repeated.

Greek medicine, I continued, did not come straight to us, to Western Europe, from the Greeks. The Arabs inherited the legacy of ancient Greece and valued it for what it was—the accumulated knowledge of centuries, but a knowledge that did very little good in its original Greek. It had to be translated in Arabic, the lingua franca of its day.

They, too, had problems and *elephas* (true leprosy) was one of them. The description of leprosy, described in unmistakable terms, they understood, but the name was all wrong. The Arabs already had elephantiasis, which they called *das fil.* This was true elephantiasis, characterized by swollen, wrinkled, thick-skinned, elephantine legs, another of the world's "common" diseases that I never see.

The Arab translators knew that *elephas* was not *das fil.* Leprosy was not elephantiasis. They were two separate diseases and therefore, needed separate names. So they picked a word, *Juzam.* Thus, *elephas* (modern leprosy) of ancient Greek writers became *Juzam.*

The next step in the transmission of ancient knowledge was for the lingua franca of the Arab world to be translated into the lingua franca of the European world, Latin. And here's where the confusion came in. *Juzam* in Arabic became *lepra* in Latin. That word was not picked by theologians but by doctors, often Jewish doctors, who shared both cultures but, of course, never read the Septuagint, except in the original Hebrew. To them, *sara'at* was *sara'at,* not *lepra,* but to Western Europeans, *sara'at* didn't exist. *Lepra* (in Greek) was a disease of ritual uncleanliness. *Lepra* (in Latin) was a specific disease, leprosy. And *lepra* was *lepra.*

And lepers had to live "without the camp." In a single stroke, a word chosen as a descriptive term covering a vague collection of ritual problems became changed, and a specific disease of no religious significance became a curse. And what a curse. During the Middle Ages, those pronounced as suffering from "leprosy" had the funeral rites of the dead performed for them. Their property was usually confiscated, and they were excluded from inhabited towns.

Like these lepers, Mrs. Dastur considered her life finished. She was a leper. And even if she was from India, she was a Christian. Her family had been Christians for generations and her attitude toward her own disease was the legacy of an attitude that had been imposed on medieval Europe by its universal Church and carried on by both the Church and popular folklore. Lepers were to be given "cup and clapper," a bowl into which to receive alms and a noisemaker to warn others of their coming. And each leper became known by the biblical name, *Lazar.*

That too, was a jumble of linguistic and religious confusion. Lazarus was a beggar covered with sores. In the parable, he lay at the rich man's gate, but only apocryphally was he given the diagnosis of leprosy. This unfounded diagnosis was widespread: Many leper hospitals on the continent of Europe were dedicated to St. Lazarus; an order of chivalry, the Knights of St. Lazarus, separated from the Knights hospitalers in the late eleventh century to devote themselves to the welfare of lepers; hospitals for lepers were widely referred to as lazar houses.

Lazarus, the undiagnosed leper, was only the beginning of confusion. By some strange and tortuous thinking, Lazarus the beggar became identified with Lazarus of Bethany, whom Jesus raised from the dead. This may have given the lepers some hope at least, for it seemed to promise certain resurrection to the lepers.

But none of this was helping my leper. She had "the same curse, the same affliction."

I was falling into her trap. She didn't have leprosy. I knew that. I told her again.

"What do I have?"

I wasn't certain.

That did little to increase her confidence in my diagnostic acumen. At least I did know what part of her nervous system was diseased. It was not her nerves. It was not the nerves of the skin that were not carrying messages. Those nerves were working fine. Her disease was in the spinal cord, where the nerve fibers carrying pain

99

from the hand segregated themselves from nerves carrying other sensations from the hand to the brain.

"Not my nerves?" she asked.

"No."

"Not leprosy?"

"No."

"Something else?"

"Yes."

"Like what?"

I hate listing possible diagnoses. I don't want patients to worry about unlikely possibilities. I had no choice. "A cyst of the spinal cord." That was the most likely one.

"What else?"

"A tumor."

"Cancer?"

That was possible.

She smiled. To her, that would be better than leprosy.

"How do we find out?"

We would start with a myelogram, an X-ray of her spinal cord. It would show us if her cord was swollen by a cyst or a tumor.

She nodded. That was what we would do.

Mrs. Dastur was admitted to the hospital the next day and two days later she underwent a myelogram. Her spinal cord was enlarged. It was more likely a cyst than a tumor, but to be certain she'd need surgery. If it was a tumor, the surgeon would take a small biopsy and then we'd see if it was malignant or not and decide if a course of radiation therapy would be indicated. If it were a cyst, the surgeon would drain it.

Would she get better?

Perhaps.

More important, we'd know what she had. And the drain would keep her from getting any worse. With a drain in it, the cyst would no longer expand.

The next day she had her operation. The surgeon found a cyst and put in a drain.

I met her right outside the operating room as she was just waking up and told her the good news. No tumor. No cancer. A cyst.

Was I certain?

I was.

Would she get better?

She'd get no worse.

"My leprosy?" she asked.

"You don't have leprosy," I reassured her. She was discharged a week later, unchanged.

I saw her four weeks later. She was unchanged, as she should have been. She was no better and absolutely no worse.

And so it went for six months, until she could no longer restrain herself.

"Why are you lying to me?" she demanded.

"Lying?"

"Leprosy."

"But you don't . . . ."

"I do."

"You had a cyst."

"I am no better."

"We told you you might not get any better."

She was again unimpressed.

We argued. She needed proof. She was a mathematician. The surgeon said he saw a cyst. He had done no biopsy. No one had looked at her tissues. We'd done no tests. It was leprosy.

"But you're no worse."

"Leprosy moves very slowly at times."

I had to prove to her that she didn't have leprosy. Proving that a patient doesn't have a particular disease is not that easy. Diagnostic medicine as a discipline is designed to prove what a patient has, not what he or she does not have. The latter is very difficult. At times, almost impossible. Absence of positive proof is not proof of absence. I had no choice. I had to give it my best shot.

I ordered an electromyogram with nerve conduction tests of both arms. Leprosy was a disease of nerves. It prevented the nerves from conducting their messages. A nerve conduction velocity would show me that her nerves were able to conduct messages at a normal rate. More important, I could show the results to her. And they would be a set of numbers. A mathematician should understand them.

I ordered it.

She took the test.

It was normal. All of the nerves of her right arm were normal. Intact. Uninjured. Able to carry normal electrical impulses at a normal rate of speed. No leprosy.

And not enough proof for Mrs. Dastur. "Absence of proof," she reminded me, "is not proof of absence."

I did not know what else to do. I tried explaining everything to her yet once again, hoping to impress her with the power of my logic. It didn't work. I was trying to protect her from her fate.

That night at home, I read about the history of leprosy. I hadn't meant to, but I had trouble concentrating on anything else. Here was a patient I couldn't help because I could not prove to her that she didn't have a disease that she didn't have.

So I read about leprosy. Not in southern India. That would have just increased my sense of helplessness. European leprosy. The leprosy of saga and folklore. The leprosy of Scandinavia, where leprosy took a firm stronghold and held out for longer than it did in other parts of Europe. I read about the men who studied leprosy. And the man who isolated the cause of leprosy, Armauer Hansen. And his teacher and mentor, D. C. Danielssen. Danielssen saw some rods in the nerves and skin of patients with leprosy. These, he thought, might be bacteria. "Degenerating fat" is what the leading German pathologist Virchow called them. It was Hansen who proved they were bacteria and that leprosy was a bacterial disease. He discovered a way to stain the bacillus, Hansen's bacillus, and prove it was there.

Or not there.

If numbers didn't work, perhaps a picture would.

I called a friend who was a dermatologist. He saw Mrs. Dastur for me and performed several skin biopsies on her and stained them for Hansen's bacillus.

There was no bacillus in any of the biopsies. No evidence of leprosy.

He gave me the slides and I showed them to Mrs. Dastur.

She was finally impressed. The pictures worked where the numbers had failed. This was proof of absence. The bacilli weren't there. She did not have leprosy.

This was all eighteen years ago. Mrs. Dastur is seventy-five now and retired and still comes to see me once every six months.

She is no better.

And no worse.

But her leprosy has never come back.

10

SEPARATED IN TIME AND SPACE

Being a doctor has taught me a lot about directing . . . .You're doing the same thing. You're reconstructing the manifold of behavior to the point where an audience says, "Yes, that's exactly like people I know."

Jonathan Miller, MD

There is a difficulty in considering David Simpson to have been a patient of mine. I only saw him twice as a neurologist, and he certainly never agreed that he would be my patient or that I would be his doctor. The first time was almost a decade ago; the second almost about six or seven years later. David was a general surgeon who specialized in cancer surgery, especially cancer of the breast. I was a senior medical student and was working part time in the cancer research laboratory trying to develop a method to detect spread of cancer to the brain by examining the spinal fluid. The research never amounted to very much. In fact, the project was a bust.

I would see him around the hospital from time to time first during my internship and residency and then even less often as I became a practicing neuologist. Then I was asked to serve on a search committee for a new chairman of Anesthesiology. Whenever there is a need to appoint a new chairperson our medical school does what virtually every other university and medical school in the United States does. The dean names a search committee to search out the best candidate and then the dean negotiates with that candidate and if all of the negotiations go well, appoints him or her to the position. The search committee is made up primarily of individuals who represent different constituencies within the medical school that have a vested interest in the activities of the new chairperson. David Simpson, who by then was associate chairperson of the Department of General Surgery as well as director of the Section of Surgical Oncology, had an obvious interest in any new chairman of Anesthesiology. The departments of Surgery and Anesthesiology have to work together hand and glove (no pun intended). I was on the committee as a representative, not of Neurology, but of Pharmacology, where I also have an appointment. In our curriculum, the Department of Anesthesia has an obligation to teach the medical students about anesthesia and pain-killing medicines within the courses directed by the Pharmacology Department. Hence we had a vested interest and there I was, attending meetings every second week for almost nine months.

As I left the last meeting, David stopped me. We were on a first-name basis by then. He asked me to come by his office for a minute. Once we were there, he told me he'd like my opinion on a medical problem he had, a neurologic problem. I told him I'd be glad to but I had two conditions. I would tell him exactly what I thought. No beating around the bush. No euphemisms.

That was precisely what he wanted. What was the other condition?

"A doctor-patient relationship requires one doctor and one patient. In ours, I am going to be the doctor and you're going to be the patient. Period. If you're going to be the doctor, the relationship is over since I will not be the patient."

He agreed completely.

The story was not a complicated one. About ten years earlier he'd had an episode of retrobulbar neuritis.

"Damn," I said to myself. "Damn, damn, damn. A disease I cannot cure."

One morning as soon as his eyes were opened, he realized that something was wrong with his vision. He closed his left eye and everything looked normal. He closed his right eye and everything in front of him was blurred. Things on either side looked pretty good, but in the center his vision was fuzzy. No, worse than fuzzy. He went into the bathroom and looked at his face in the mirror using only his left eye. The middle of his face was a dark blur. No nose. No eyes, fuzzy cheeks, a fuzzy forehead, but his ears were sharp as could be.

He went to see a friend of his who was an opthalmologist. The opthalmologist examined him, did some tests, and told him he had retrobulbar neuritis.

David knew what that meant. Retrobulbar neuritis is inflammation in the optic nerve carrying visual images from the eye toward the brain. That inflammation was located just behind the globe or bulb of his left eye; hence the name. He also knew that the inflammation did not directly involve the nerve fibers themselves. So it wasn't true neuritis. The inflammation involved the lining of the nerves, the insulation, a layer surrounding each nerve fiber, made up of a fatty substance called myelin. Retrobulbar neuritis means inflammation of the myelin. A disease of the myelin, and he knew only one disease of myelin. Multiple sclerosis.

He asked the ophthalmologist if he had MS.

"No," his friend told him.

Would he get it?

"Don't worry about that. You're not going to get MS," his friend reassured him.

On what basis could the opthalmologist have said that, I wondered. Not science. Not epidemiology. At least a third of such patients go on to get MS, most within less than a decade. Friendship, I concluded. Friendship and the usual tendency among doctors to tell each other reassuring white lies.

David had then asked his friend if there was any treatment.

Steroids might help, but he'd recover without them.

David declined the steroids and in six weeks his retrobulbar neuritis had cleared. His vision was back to normal. He felt certain that the story was over.

I was certain that it wasn't. If it were, there would have been no reason at all for me to be there in his office listening to any of this. "MS." I thought to myself. "Why did it have to be MS?"

MS means multiple areas of sclerosis or scarring in the brain and spinal cord. Each of these scars represents an area of inflammation; inflammation of the myelin, hence the euphemism demyelinating disease. Clinically you diagnose MS by history and neurologic examination, but primarily by history. Most often the examination merely confirms the history and the various tests we do add further confirmation. To have MS, the patient must have multiple areas of involvement of the brain or spinal cord and these must be separated in time; that is, they must occur at different times, first one, then another, then a third. They must also be separated in space. They must be in different places in the nervous system, the optic nerve, right smack behind the eye, then the cerebellum perhaps, at the back of the brain, or the brain stem connecting the brain to the spinal cord, then the other eye or the spinal cord itself.

"Separated in time and space."

Four years later, he told me, he started having some trouble in the operating room. Four years—separated in time.

What kind of trouble?

His left hand felt clumsy.

Weak?

No. Clumsy. Uncoordinated. He had trouble doing two-handed sutures.

Cerebellar involvement. That meant that his second episode had involved a far different spot in his brain. The second criterion had been fulfilled. Separation in space.

It only lasted three weeks. Maybe four. He tried not to think about it. Perhaps he'd been too tired. Perhaps he'd had a pinched nerve. He had not seen anyone about it. No neurologist. Not even his friend the ophthalmologist.

A year and a half later, he started having trouble walking. Year and a half. Another separation in time.

What kind of trouble? Was it an imbalance? A sort of clumsiness?

Such imbalance or clumsiness would mean that his cerebellar difficulties had returned.

"No." He had not been clumsy. He had not lost his sense of balance. His legs had been stiff.

Both legs?

Yes.

A third place. The spinal cord. Another separation in space. Clinically, historically, the most likely diagnosis was MS. David Simpson handed me several sheets of paper. They were laboratory reports from one of the other medical schools in Chicago. The name of the patient was Power, not Simpson. The reports were of various tests on spinal fluid.

I looked at Simpson. "Yours?" I asked.

"Mine," he replied.

I have no idea who performed the spinal taps and where. I didn't need that information so I didn't ask and Simpson didn't offer any such information. According to the lab reports, two spinal taps had been done well over a year apart; the more recent one just a few months before. Analysis of spinal fluid obtained from such spinal taps never prove that a patient has MS. Then why do we do them? Two reasons. The first is to make sure there is no evidence of any other disease that might alter the content of the spinal fluid. Many such diseases would cause far greater elevations of protein or white-cell counts than we see in MS. The protein would reflect injury to nerve cells themselves while the white blood count would reflect active infection. Power's results—Simpson's results—showed no such changes. The protein levels were normal both times. Both times the white blood cell counts were just slightly elevated.

The second reason for looking at the spinal fluid is to see if any abnormalities can be found that support the diagnosis. MS seems to involve some sort of immunologic change, an immune reaction against the myelin. In this immune reaction antibodies are formed in the brain and appear in the spinal fluid. Both times, his spinal fluid showed such antibodies. Both times, the analysis supported the historical impression that immune reactions were going on in the brain or spinal cord.

"Supportive evidence," I said.

"I know."

Next he showed me a CAT scan. Again, it had some other name on it. Strickland, I think. It was normal. It often is in MS. Then why do we do them? We used to do them to make sure we weren't being fooled. To make sure we weren't missing some other, treatable diagnosis. Today we do MRI scans. They not only give negative evidence showing the absence of other significant diseases; they also supply positive evidence, showing the exact areas of myelin injury, the precise location of inflammation, of the plaques of scarring, the multiple regions of sclerosis. Injuries scattered in place. And if you do more than one, separated by months or years, you also see areas of involvement separated in time.

Simpson handed me the MRI scan.

I looked at it. The name on it was Boone. The lesions were there. Behind the eye. In the brain. In the brain stem. At least a dozen of them.

"MS," I said.

"That's what you think?"

"MS," I repeated. "The possibilities that this is anything else are two. Remote and none. And I'd bet on none."

"You're pretty sure?"

"As sure as I can ever be with MS," I told him. I then talked to him about MS itself. Telling him that the course was quite variable, that the prognosis was not universally bad, that many patients remained active for many years, for decades even.

"As surgeons?" he asked.

He was right. He needed more than average control of his movements. Any disability at all in hand control and he could no longer operate. He could become disabled much more easily than a lawyer,

107

or an accountant, or a banker, or a secretary, or a receptionist, or almost anyone except perhaps a diamond cutter.

"Can you cure me?"

"There are no cures," I told him.

He knew that. "Can you prevent the next attack?" he asked.

I gave him as complete an answer as I could. The bottom line was no. We talked about research that was going on with various drugs that suppress the immune system. None had been shown to prevent the development of any new areas of demyelinization, of new sclerosis, or of new loss of nerve function. In fact, it was not clear that they helped at all.

"But it is an immune disorder, isn't it?"

"Yes, but a strange one. The immune response occurs not in lymph nodes or bursae or the other homes of the immune system, but in the brain itself. Very strange."

Simpson shook his head. "But I can cure cancer," he said. "I'm a surgeon." I told him that he should see me on a regular basis, like any other patient, and he nodded. "In my office, perhaps."

He never came to my office to see me. I knew that he wouldn't. The name on the spinal fluid was not his. Nor the CAT scan. Nor the MRI. In his mind, no one could ever see him in a neurologist's office. There could be no rumors. No suspicions. He was a surgeon. He cured cancer.

I did see him around the hospital from time to time and also at other committee meetings. Medical schools thrive on committees and committee meetings. I don't. Neither did he, so we only ran into each other at such conclaves irregularly. Sometimes I would see him walking down a hallway, dragging one leg, or the other, or neither or even both. The attacks obviously came and went but some left scattered traces of loss. At meetings, I could sometimes detect changes in his speech. Slurring of his syllables. Then three months later his speech would be almost normal. Almost but not quite.

I never saw him in the operating room, but I heard rumors. Nothing very substantive. A mild tremor. Pressure? Nerves? Drinking? A little clumsiness. More pressure. More drinking? No, the tremors were gone. The rumor mill had no idea what was going on. And he was still a hell of a fine surgeon.

Then one morning as I was letting myself into my office—it was before eight, no secretaries had yet arrived, no receptionists—I got a phone call from one of my residents. David Simpson had just been admitted to the hospital, to Neurology, to be my patient.

"MS," I said sadly.

"Brain abscesses," she said, correcting me.

"He couldn't have had brain abscesses all these years."

"These are new," she said.

And I knew what had happened. He was a surgeon. He could cure cancer. The impatience of watching and waiting had not been for him. He had sought some other doctor who was willing to use immunosuppressive drugs. And they had worked not on his MS so much but on his ability to ward off infection and now he was paying the price with secondary infections. Opportunistic infection—infections that only happen because the immune system isn't working. Like an AIDS patient. A sort of iatrogenic form of AIDS.

"What's he been on?"

She gave me a list. He'd been on every immunosuppressive agent as well as every anticancer drug that caused immunosuppression that I'd ever heard of. And not just one at a time, but combination therapies. Two, three at a time. What damn-fool neurologist was treating him? There was no evidence that regimes like that did any good in MS. In cancer, yes. Then I knew. No neurologist was treating him. He cured cancer. He knew about anticancer drugs in combined protocols. Two at a time, or more. And he was treating himself.

"Who's his doctor?"

"You are," was the answer.

"Not now. Who's been giving him all those damn drugs?"

"He says you're the only neurologist he's ever seen."

He'd been his own doctor. He'd not only treated himself; he'd experimented on himself.

I went across to the Neurology floor. The resident, Garcia, showed me the MRI scan. Simpson had well over a dozen abscesses. She then told me what antibiotics he was on. Hopefully they would work.

Dave Simpson was in a private room. The room was dark. He had an IV running. There was a respirator at his bedside just in case. It seems he also had developed pneumonia.

"Why?" I started to ask him.

He never let me finish my question.

"I'm a surgeon. Hell, I can cure cancer. Beating this should have been easy."

David Simpson, MD, associate chairman of the Department of Surgery, died three days later. The official cause of death was listed as multiple cerebral abscesses due to chronic immunosuppression, a classic iatrogenic—physician caused—illness. That word *iatrogenic* never appeared on the death certificate, nor did *self-experimentation,* but it was those two conditions that had led to his death. He had never become too disabled to operate and no one had learned that he had MS so that no well-founded rumors had blunted his career. He had merely died of it all. But had all those drugs he'd taken made any difference? I'll never know. No one ever will. It was an experiment with only one subject, a subject with a disease which has a remarkably variable and unpredictable course. There had been no control subjects and no objective observers at all. Merely the subject acting as observer while the observer became the subject, a process that prevented any rational understanding and measurement of what was actually happening to his disease— and to his entire body—for that matter.

His life was cut short far too early by his inability to deal with the reality of what he had and then trying to cope with that within a doctor-patient relationship just like any other patient.

And being a surgeon was no excuse. Or was it? John Hunter, the father of modern surgery in the United Kingdom, had done the same thing two centuries before. Hunter (1728–1793) was a Scotsman whose older brother William Hunter (1718–1783) was a great anatomist and clinician in London. John Hunter moved to London to work with his older brother. He showed considerable skill in dissection while working in his brother's dissection rooms. He demonstrated the branches of the olfactory nerves and also previously unknown branches of the fifth nerve. He was able to show the course of the arteries of the pregnant uterus and the presence of lymphatic vessels in birds. John felt that he received inadequate credit from his brother and they became estranged. Hunter then joined the army in 1760 and received considerable experience operating on gunshot wounds. He began his practice as a surgeon in 1763 and continued to lecture on anatomy and surgery in London. He soon became a noted teacher and attracted a group of brilliant pupils who later became famous, and his reputation as an anatomist, naturalist, and investigator spread rapidly.

One of his most remarkable experiments was one that he performed on himself. The question he wanted to answer was whether syphilis and gonorrhea were separate stages of the same disease or two separate diseases. Today, of course, armed by a century of careful bacteriologic study, the answer is so obvious that the question seems preposterous; hardly scientific at all. But that was not the case in the 1780s. It was a hotly debated issue; after all, human nature hasn't changed that much and these two disorders often kept each other company.

Hunter described his experiment and the results in *A Treatise on the Venereal Disease,* which was first published in 1786. John Hunter believed that he had proved that the two disorders were but one single disease, a hypothesis he had accepted even before his experiment. In the experiment he obtained pus from a patient with gonorrhea. He then scarified his penis with a lancet dipped in the pus. This was in May 1767. A swollen gland soon popped up in his right groin but he never developed gonorrhea. Later, secondary syphilis showed up in the form of a rash and of an abscess on one of his tonsils. The sores on the penis he treated with mercury-containing ointments, and for the other manifestations he rubbed other mercurial ointment into his legs with a view to modifying the disease but not to completely curing it. Finally, about three years after the beginning of his experiment, he rubbed in much more ointment in order to cure himself of the disease. He was convinced that he had confirmed his hypothesis. There was only one venereal disease, "*the* venereal disease." Not two. He had given himself pus from a patient with gonorrhea and had come away from the experience with syphilis.

What had gone wrong?

Why was he so off base?

Remember, this was long before Louis Pasteur and Robert Koch and the rise of bacteriology. Bacteria were not seen, identified, and cultured. Koch's postulates could not even have been fantasized, much less relied upon. There are several problems. First, it is obvious to us that the donor of the pus had syphilis. There was no way for Hunter to know that. There were no blood tests for syphilis then. To Hunter the diagnosis of syphilis required visible evidence—a site of chancre infection on the skin of the penis. The infamous chancre. But such chancres can be hidden from sight. They can lurk inside the urethra itself. Without bacteriologic identification of the spirochete of syphilis, a process not developed until this century, that could not have been accomplished.

Why didn't Hunter get both gonorrhea and syphilis? The answer is not quite so clear. The donor had pus. Syphilis does not produce pus. The commonest cause of such pus is gonorrhea. Ergo, the donor had both. But did he? Again we don't know. It is not uncommon for chancres of syphilis to become secondarily infected and for that secondary infection to produce pus. Such secondary infections are not contagious. So it is very possible that the donor only had syphilis and all that Hunter demonstrated was the venereal spread of syphilis, a fact that had been known from the inception of the disease.

On the other hand, it is more likely that the donor had both diseases but virtually no disease is 100 percent infective. Not everyone who comes in contact with a patient with the flu gets flu. Some do, some don't—and for lots of reasons. The same is true for every other disease including syphilis, gonorrhea, and AIDS.

So it was an experiment that was bound to fail. It was an attempt to answer a question that for technical reasons could not yet be answered. It's a good thing he did it to himself and not some innocent volunteer.

Or was it?

Years later he developed cardiac pain, angina pectoris, and then died of an acute myocardial death. In the l790s and well into this century syphilis was a well-known cause of cardiac disease. In the third stage, syphilis attacks the aorta as it leaves the heart, resulting in angina, heart failure, and death. Over the years, most writers who pondered the question concluded that the cardiac pain, from which Hunter suffered for years, and ultimately his death were caused by syphilis.

So perhaps David Simpson was merely following his surgical heritage. Self-experimentation leading to an iatrogenic death. Unfortunately, it cannot be romanticized in quite that way.

More careful reviews of the well-described autopsy of John Hunter have shown that his angina and death were due to plain old-fashioned atherosclerotic coronary artery disease—high blood pressure, cholesterol stress, type A personality.

There was nothing old-fashioned about David Simpson's death.

TO TREAT OR NOT TO TREAT

The art of medicine consists of amusing the patient while nature cures the disease.

Voltaire

The clinical problem was straightforward enough. The patient was a young woman who was about to become engaged to a doctor, one of my residents. That is how she all but became one of my patients. I never saw her as a patient, so of course, I never examined her. I did however discuss her neurologic problem with her fiance-to-be. Or, to put it in the proper perspective, he discussed her problem with me. He told me her history and the results of her neurologic examination and asked for confirmation of what he had done—not as simple a request as he had assumed it to be.

She was twenty-seven. She had her MBA and a job in a large advertising firm in Chicago, a job that included a lot of contact with clients, a job in which her looks, personality, and public appearance were not insignificant. She was quite a looker. Such considerations are supposed to be a thing of the past, but so far are not. I had met her once or twice socially, at departmental receptions and the like. She dressed in a way that made it impossible not to notice her thin waist, well-tapered legs, and her pale white face outlined by long, glimmering black hair. It was the face that stood out.

The day before, according to her fiancé, she'd been in perfect health. Her usual buoyant self. Then at about two o'clock the right side of her face had felt strange. It was hard for her to describe it much better than that. It wasn't numb. It didn't tingle. There was no pain. No discomfort. Yet it didn't feel right. She looked in a mirror. She looked normal. Thank God.

The feeling persisted, intensified. She checked again and her face still looked normal in her mirror. As long as her mirror was already out, she decided to touch up her lipstick. She puckered her lips. They didn't pucker normally; the right corner hardly moved. That was strange; more than strange. It was downright peculiar.

Within half an hour, the entire right side of her face was paralyzed. Nothing moved. Not her right eyebrow. Not her right cheek. Nothing. She panicked: my God, what was happening to her? A stroke? Her grandmother had had a stroke, at eighty-one years old. She was only twenty-seven. She was too young to have a stroke. Or was she? John, her fiancé and my resident, had told her about patients with blocked vessels to their brains that ruptured. Patients his age. Patients her age. She wasn't too young.

Panic.

She called John. She was frightened. She told him what had happened.

"It's probably a Bell's palsy."

"What's that?"

"Some inflammation of the nerve to your face."

"Not a stroke?"

"No."

"Thank God!"

She took a cab to the hospital, already much relieved, and met John, who then examined her. All he found was a complete paralysis of all of the muscles of the right half of her face. These muscles are all controlled by a single nerve. Everything else was functioning normally. Her tongue, the muscles that moved her jaw, those that moved her eyes, her ability to feel sensations such as touch, temperature, the prick of a pin. All that was intact. Normal.

The diagnosis was as he had expected. An acute, sudden paralysis of the seventh nerve, a Bell's palsy, named after the English physician who first described the disorder.

He told her the diagnosis once again.

Was he certain?

He was.

Absolutely?

Yes, but they could get a CAT scan to be certain.

They did that and the CAT scan was normal. No brain tumor. No stroke. No ruptured blood vessels.

Relief.

A deep sigh. A few tears of relief. Then the questions. What was Bell's palsy?

Inflammation of the seventh nerve on one side of the face.

What caused it?

No one knew for sure. Perhaps a viral infection. There was always a great deal of swelling of the nerve itself.

What would happen to her? Would her face always be paralyzed?

No.

Would she recover?

Yes.

One hundred percent? Back to normal?

Probably.

Only probably? What did that mean?

Ten to twenty percent of the patients ended up with some mild weakness.

What did that mean?

The face would almost look normal.

Almost?

Especially when it wasn't moving, but . . . .

But what?

She might have some trouble closing her eye. Or puckering her lips tightly. That, he joked, might bother him more than her.

The humor was lost on her. She knew there had to be something he wasn't telling her. She asked the questions she'd been trained to ask. What was the worst-case scenario?

Total paralysis. No recovery.

How often?

Four percent.

One out of twenty-five!

Maybe less.

One out of twenty-five! She couldn't go through life like that. It would kill her. Her job. Her life. Her whole life. A freak. There had to be something he could do. He was a doctor. He was a neurologist. This was a neurologic problem.

Do something!

Do anything!

There had to be a treatment of some sort. Wasn't there any treatment for Bell's palsy? Any way to decrease the swelling and inflammation? Any way to keep her from being deformed for the rest of her life?

Yes, there was.

What?

Large doses of steroids.

"Well then, give them to me. Help me. Save me."

He gave her a prescription and now he was asking me to tell him that he'd done the right thing. That was going to be hard for me to do. He had first and foremost broken a cardinal rule of medicine, one of those unwritten laws that some people are never smart enough to obey: Never treat people with whom you are emotionally involved. Never. No parents, children, siblings, spouses, sweethearts, lovers, best friends. If they come to you, pick the best doctor available and then stay out of it. Completely out of it.

The role of steroids was far from proved. Some people felt they helped in Bell's palsy, others didn't. She pushed. And he made a treatment decision. He knew how much her facial appearance meant to her. He had to help her, to prevent her from being deformed for the rest of her life.

I told him a story. It had taken place about fifteen years earlier. I'd been about his age. I was a neurologist in the army then. A major came in to see me; he'd noted a funny feeling in his face half an hour earlier.

I examined him. He had an acute Bell's palsy. I told him about his disease.

Was there any treatment?

I told him about the use of steroids. I described the equivocal results and the side effects.

"So what did you do?"

"I gave him a prescription for a one-week course of prednisone and told him to come back in one week. After all, if steroids ever worked, they should work better when started early and here I had a chance to start them within a couple of hours of the onset of the Bell's palsy."

"I did the right thing," John said with obvious relief.

I made no direct reply. "In one week he returned and he was normal. Absolutely normal. Bell's usually takes months to recover. Often a year or more. One week and he was back to normal. Of course, most patients didn't get steroids that quickly."

John was beaming. He'd done the right thing. His fiancée had started the prednisone within hours of the onset of her Bell's palsy. It would help. She'd recover. He'd saved her.

I, too, had felt triumphant. I, too, had helped a patient. I, too, had beamed.

"Say Doc," the major said, "do you still want me to take this medicine?"

"What medicine?" I sputtered.

"This medicine." He reached into his pocket to get his bottle of prednisone tablets, I assumed. No bottle appeared. No tablets. No pills. Instead, a prescription. My prescription. The prescription.

"These pills of yours. Do you still want me to take them? If you do, I'll have to go to the pharmacy. I was too busy last week."

Too busy? He'd never gotten the prescription filled. He'd never taken any prednisone. He'd gotten better on his own. Unless the mere threat of treatment had been sufficient, and I was skeptical of that.

"Well, Doc?" he had persisted.

"No," I said.

"So I shouldn't have given her steroids," John said dejectedly.

"That's not the point," I said. "It should not have been your decision."

"Why not?" he asked.

I told him why not.

He was not convinced. He'd made the best decision. He'd done what was best for her.

Without any nonmedical considerations?

Yes.

Was he confident of that?

Yes. Absolutely so.

Did he give everyone steroids for Bell's palsy? Absolutely everyone?

Yes. No. No, not really.

So what was the difference?

She was so beautiful.

Did that mean that only the beautiful should not be disfigured?

Of course not. That's not what he meant and I knew it.

I knew no such thing. We were at an impasse.

John's fiancée-to-be did not get better in a week. Or in a month. After six months she started to improve. By the end of a year she had regained most of her function. Most, but not all. At rest, her face was back to normal, but her smile was just a bit crooked. She could not close her right eye completely and her ability to pucker her lips was far from normal. That was the way it stayed. Not normal, but far from grotesque.

John never married her. Or she never married him. No one told me which until she introduced herself to me almost a decade later at a party. She was married and juggling a career, a husband, and two children with great artistry and imagination.

She told me her name and smiled. To a neurologist, the diagnosis was obviously an old Bell's palsy on the right. I, of course, said nothing.

"I was once engaged to a resident of yours," she began. "Then I got Bell's palsy."

A light flashed in my memory.

"What happened?"

"He couldn't adjust. At first, I thought it was me. I had to look perfect. A Pepsodent smile. Thin waist. Long legs, a perfect face. That was me. If not, I'd die. Then a Bell's palsy. Paralysis of half my face. And I was still me. I was still clever, and bright, a good businesswoman, and a loving partner for life. Except he didn't see it that way. He wanted me to be better. He needed me to. I had to be his perfect showpiece. He kept me on steroids for five months. Hell, no one does that. He cared more about my pucker than about me. It wasn't me. It was him. I dumped him. What ever happened to him?"

"He's in practice."

"Where?"

"California. LA."

"That figures." She turned to walk over to the buffet. She had done the right thing. Had I? Had I? I thought I had. A student's failure to learn is not always due to the teacher's shortcomings. It only feels that way to the teacher.

PART THREE

CALL IT RESEARCH

The only difference between Johns Hopkins and your medical school [The University of Illinois] is that at Hopkins most of the lousy teachers do world-class research.

A Fellow Intern

12

SUCH IS FAME

The best scientist is open to experience and begins with romance—the idea that anything is possible.

Ray Bradbury

Fame was the farthest thing from Roberta Rose Richards' mind when she came to see me for the first time. She did not want fame or fortune. It was good health she was after; the ability to get out of an overstuffed easy chair by herself or out of a car, to walk through a door without shuffling, to be able to cut her own meat in less than ten minutes, to be able to fasten her own bra. To feel like herself, not an old woman who soon would be no longer able to care for herself. She needed to be able to do that, to have a sense of well-being.

She had been referred to me by a neurologist at the Mayo Clinic, where she had been going for her medical care for fifteen years. They were the ones who had made the diagnosis of Parkinson's disease and begun her on levodopa, but that miracle of modern medicine had not helped her. The physicians at the Mayo Clinic had also discovered her hyperthyroid condition and removed her thyroid gland, but that they'd done fifteen years earlier. Her Parkinson's disease was the problem now and they were not helping that. She was getting worse. Slower. More disabled. Each time she traveled from Muncie, Indiana, to Rochester, Minnesota, it was more difficult for her.

Was there anything more they could do to help her? The neurologist didn't think so. Perhaps, he suggested, it might be easier on her if she didn't have to come so far for her medical care.

Was there anyone he could recommend? Someone who knew about Parkinson's disease?

There was, but the doctor was in Chicago.

That was all right with her. Fifty miles was a lot better than five hundred.

So Roberta Rose Richards became my patient, my challenge.

And a challenge she was, from the very beginning. Her records arrived from the Mayo Clinic several days before she came in for her first office visit. I read them through and had my plan of attack outlined in my mind before I ever saw her. She was described as a patient with classic Parkinson's disease who had not responded at all to levodopa and on whom the doctors at the Mayo Clinic had essentially given up. They could do no more.

I was sure I could. Parkinson's disease was my forte. Patients with Parkinson's disease, in my experience, always responded to levodopa. They all improved unless they didn't really have Parkinson's disease, or they developed side effects from the medicine, or they had some other medical condition that interfered with the treatment in some way. That's as it should be. Parkinson's disease is due to the loss of a specific chemical in the brain known as dopamine, normally made by a specific set of nerve cells called the *substantia nigra*. These neurons manufacture dopamine, which in turn acts as a message courier or neurotransmitter and allows the substantia nigra to control one of the major motor areas of the brain, the striatum. The dopamine made by the cells of the substantia nigra acts upon the cells of the striatum. If there is no dopamine to act on the receptors of the striatal nerve cells, the patient develops Parkinson's disease. But the striatum is normal. If the lost messenger is replaced, the patient improves. That's what levodopa does. It enters the striatum, is transformed into dopamine, and acts on the normal dopamine receptors of the striatum.

A return to normalcy. Not all the way, but a darn sight closer than Mrs. Richards had ever gotten.

I was going to succeed where the Mayo Clinic had failed. She'd get better or at least I'd know the reason why. After all, I'd been treating patients with Parkinson's disease for four years. I was an expert.

As she walked into my office, I was ready. I had already formulated the questions I had to answer. Did she really have Parkinson's disease? After all, if she had some other neurologic disease, the medicine should not be expected to work. That was step one.

Step two would be to determine if she had really been a levodopa failure. Just because one neurologist said she was didn't make it true, even if he was from the Mayo Clinic. Being a neurologist at the Mayo Clinic didn't make someone an expert on Parkinson's disease. And many neurologists used levodopa too gingerly, in doses that were too small, and compounded that by stopping too soon. Too little for not long enough. Had she taken enough for long enough and still not improved?

Or had her response been limited by side effects? If so, I had a new experimental drug that might eliminate those side effects. They hadn't tried her on that in Rochester, Minnesota.

And if all that yielded no results, I even knew what other diseases to look for. Hypothyroidism. A normal level of thyroid activity is needed for the brain cells to function normally. She'd had thyroid surgery fifteen years before. She was taking replacement therapy. Perhaps she needed more.

I was ready for her, as ready as any one doctor had ever been for one patient.

At the appointed hour on the appointed day, Ms. Roberta Rose Richards came shuffling into my office, looking just like every other Parkinson's patient I have ever diagnosed. She had the same tremor, the same stiffness (which by convention we call rigidity), the same slowness of movement, the same imbalance, the same loss of facial expression. Everything was the same, from her slow, monotonous speech to her small, tight handwriting (what doctors call micrographia). She could have come from James Parkinson's original essay. She had what he had called "The Shaking Palsy."

And there was no evidence of anything else. No signs of any other neurologic problem. None at all. So much for step one. One point for Mayo Clinic.

On to step two. Had the treatment been adequate?

Perhaps. But only perhaps. She'd taken three grams of levodopa a day for four months. There had been occasional patients who had required more for longer for an adequate response, but most had shown some response at the dose she had taken.

Had she improved at all?

No.

Was she certain?

She was.

Had she had any side effects?

No.

Nausea?

No.

Dizziness?

No. None at all.

That meant we could try higher doses for longer. On to step three.

The physical exam showed no evidence of hypothyroidism, but

I'd been fooled before. Her last tests were six months old.

End of history and examination. On to discussion.

Could I help her?

Yes.

How?

She needed a more exhaustive trial of levodopa.

But she'd taken levodopa before and it hadn't helped.

The trial had not been adequate, I explained.

Anything else?

We would re-evaluate her thyroid condition.

They'd done that at the Mayo Clinic.

I'd like her to see an endocrinologist, I told her.

She accepted that, but wanted to know what we'd do when those ideas didn't pan out; after all, she'd taken levodopa and the doctors at the Mayo Clinic said her thyroid function was normal.

I told her about the experimental drugs I was studying. First levodopa, then the newer drugs. And also I wanted the endocrinologist to check more than her thyroid. There were other glands near the thyroid called the parathyroid glands. Sometimes they were injured during thyroid surgery and if they weren't functioning normally, that could sometimes change brain function. Even for a neurologist, that was a lot of sometimes.

I started her on levodopa and sent her off to the endocrinologist. We started at two grams a day for four weeks.

She got no better. And the endocrinologist said her thyroid function was fine. So was her parathyroid gland as far as he could tell.

Three grams a day for a month.

She got no better.

Four grams for a month.

Five grams, another month.

Six.

Seven.

Eight.

Six months had gone by. She had not improved a bit. In fact, she was certain she was getting worse. So was I. Ten grams a day was the most I'd ever used before. I got her up to twelve. At that point, we both knew it was time to try something else. Did I have something else to try?

I did.

What? ·

Newer antiparkinsonian medications.

Would they help her?

I thought they would.

Why?

Because she had Parkinson's disease.

But levodopa hadn't worked.

That was the rub. Levodopa hadn't helped her even though she took more per day than any other patient I have ever treated. But these medicines were different, I protested.

"How?" she asked me.

I explained it to her as well as I could. Levodopa was a natural substance, an amino acid, one of the building blocks of the body's proteins. She took it, it entered into her blood stream and some of it got into her brain—but in the brain levodopa does nothing unless the brain transforms it into dopamine. And for her that was probably the rub. She was probably low in both dopamine and the enzyme that makes dopamine from levodopa.

But the new medicines were different. Once they entered the brain, they were ready to go to work. They needed no enzyme to activate them. They just went right up to those waiting brain dopamine receptors and set to work, fooling the receptors into believing that they were dopamine.

She was ready to go.

So was I.

Which one, she asked.

Bromocriptine, I said.

She nodded. The name meant nothing to her.

I gave her the Patient Information Sheet and the Informed Consent Form. She read the former and signed the latter. And we got started. The usual starting dose was two and a half milligrams per day and the usual optimal dose was around forty milligrams per day. We titrated up slowly to avoid such side effects as nausea and low blood pressure. And the sky was the limit. We could go up to 160 milligrams per day: four times the average dose.

I outlined the course of therapy and gave her her medication.

"Will it help?" she asked.

"It should."

"I know, but will it?"

"I think it will." I smiled back at her.

Off she shuffled. Two and a half milligrams a day for the first week, then adding two and a half a day every Monday. In four weeks she was on ten milligrams a day and in eight weeks, she'd reached twenty milligrams a day.

Twenty was no better than ten. And ten had been no better than nothing. No response at all.

Thirty milligrams.

Forty milligrams.

Still nothing, and this was the average maintenance dose.

Fifty.

Sixty.

Eighty.

One hundred twenty.

One hundred sixty. Four times the average maintenance dose and nothing had happened. No improvement. No side effects. Just further progression of the disease.

Did I have any other tricks up my sleeve? I did. It was called lergotrile. It was a second cousin of bromocriptine. It acted in much the same way, I told her.

Why would it be better?

Some patients did better on lergotrile than on bromocriptine. And vice versa. It was impossible to predict.

She nodded. Once more she read the Patient Information Sheet and once more she signed the Informed Consent Form. And once more I gave her her instructions and the medication. And each four weeks she would trudge slowly into my office hoping against hope that I could detect some inkling of improvement she had missed. I never did. She missed nothing. She trudged on, getting slower and slower, with greater and greater imbalance.

Halfway through the lergotrile study, she tried a cane. It didn't help. By the end, she'd moved on to a walker.

Did I have any other tricks?

My bag was empty, but I couldn't give up. If she wouldn't and she hadn't yet, then neither would I. But what to do?

I went over her entire chart, starting with the first visit and my initial plan outlined with such obvious bravado. Reading it was almost painful. Three steps that had led to nothing. Did she have Parkinson's disease? Had she had any adequate trial? Was there some other factor? All had come to naught. But it had been the right plan and there was only one thing to do. Start all over again.

That's what I told her I wanted to do. I wanted to hospitalize her and make sure that we had left no stone unturned. No stone at all.

126

What did that mean?

Another visit with endocrinology. More blood tests. Skull X-rays. A spinal tap.

Why? Why did I want to do a spinal tap?

It will tell us how much dopamine your brain has lost, I began. That was an oversimplification, but not a misleading one. The spinal fluid bathes the brain and acts to carry away many of the breakdown products of the active chemicals of the brain. Dopamine is one such active chemical and its breakdown produces HVA, a normal constituent of the cerebrospinal fluid. In Parkinson's disease, the brain has less dopamine than normal and the spinal fluid, as a reflection of this, contains less HVA.

She came into the hospital. The blood tests were all normal. So were the skull X-rays. The endocrinologist found nothing; no evidence of hyperthyroidism, no evidence of hypothyroidism. We stopped her medications. This was not a step that we took lightly. It was not without risk. It was all too obvious that she had never derived any improvement from any of the medications—levodopa or the newest direct-acting agonists, bromocriptine and lergotrile—and in fact had deteriorated while taking them. But that did not mean they were doing nothing for her. Perhaps without them she would be even worse than she was. Totally immobile.

I explained that to her.

Then why must you stop them, she asked.

To study the spinal fluid.

She nodded as if she understood.

The medicines would interfere with the chemical studies we needed to make. Levodopa would increase the HVA to levels far above normal while lergotrile might either increase it or decrease it, but in either case would obscure the meaning.

She nodded again slowly, although the expression on her mask-like face had, of course, not changed.

That day I decreased her medications by half. Nothing changed. She got no worse.

I waited two days and then withdrew half of the half she was still taking, a total reduction of 75 percent. I waited for the bottom to fall out.

It didn't. Roberta didn't change at all.

Three days later I got her off everything and then, after seventy-two drug-free hours, we did her spinal tap. All of the routine chemistries were normal—just as they should be in Parkinson's disease.

127

I delivered the last sample to my lab myself and watched as my technician ran the test. A normal adult has an HVA level in the spinal fluid of between 60 and 180. A Parkinson's patient is usually below 40, often below 20, especially if the Parkinson's disease is as advanced as Roberta's.

I watched. And I waited. Science at work. I read the result as the graph paper fed out of the machine.

One hundred sixty-four.

That had to be wrong. It wasn't even borderline, much less decreased. It was at the upper limit of normal. But Roberta had Parkinson's disease, severe Parkinson's disease. And Parkinson's disease meant decreased dopamine and decreased dopamine meant decreased HVA. A simple three-part syllogism.

The technician must have screwed up. Or the machine. We needed to be absolutely certain.

He ran it again. This time I scrutinized every step. Once again I read the result as it fed out of the analyzer.

One hundred sixty-eight.

I had never seen a level that high in a patient with Parkinson's disease. And Roberta Rosa Richards had Parkinson's disease. That much I knew. I'd made the diagnosis myself with my own eyes and my own hands. I'd seen her tremor and slowness. I'd felt her rigidity. I'd seen her imbalance, her masklike face. I'd observed her micrographia. I'd heard her soft, hesitant voice. You name the manifestation of Parkinson's disease, and Roberta had it. The diagnosis was so obvious, so painfully obvious. Roberta had Parkinson's disease. Parkinson's disease with an HVA level of 164. Or 168. Take your pick.

We had to be certain. We'd do it one more time.

I took the last of her spinal fluid and ran the analysis myself. Step by step. Painstakingly referring to my own notes at each step. No master chef had ever taken more care. The three-minute procedure took almost three hours and in the end I got her HVA level.

One hundred sixty-six.

That meant she didn't have Parkinson's disease.

All you had to do was reverse the three-step syllogism.

Normal HVA meant normal dopamine and normal dopamine meant no Parkinson's disease. So Roberta Rose Richards did not have Parkinson's disease.

But what did she have?

Clinically she had Parkinson's disease. She looked like every other patient who had Parkinson's disease and did not make enough dopamine to act at the dopamine sites in the striatum. But Roberta made enough HVA. She had enough dopamine.

What did she have? Why didn't levodopa help her? Why didn't bromocriptine? Or lergotrile?

I had some ideas, but no definite answer.

If for some reason she had a disease of the striatum instead of the dopamine-producing cells of the substantia nigra, that would explain everything. If the dopamine receptor cells of the striatum were not able to respond to dopamine, she would look and act like a patient with Parkinson's disease because all of the symptoms of Parkinson's disease are due to loss of the effect of dopamine on the striatal cells.

And the HVA level would be normal. Perhaps even higher than normal as the dopamine-producing cells worked harder to produce the normal physiological balance.

And of course levodopa wouldn't work since the striatum could not respond to dopamine.

Or to bromocriptine. Or to lergotrile.

That would explain it all. But what could cause that?

I knew of two possible causes, neither of which she had. The first was hypothyroidism. In hypothyroidism, the body and the brain have decreased amounts of thyroid hormone, and without sufficient thyroid hormone the dopamine receptors of the striatum cannot respond to dopamine.

Roberta had normal levels of thyroid hormone. We'd tested them. So had the Mayo Clinic.

The other was hypoparathyroidism. In this condition the body doesn't make parathyroid hormone and without that hormone, some aspects of brain function can be changed. One of those is how the striatum responds to dopamine.

And she even had a reason to have hyporparathyroidism, a known complication of thyroid surgery.

But she didn't have hyporparathyroidism. The endocrinologists had assured me of that. Not once, but three times. Besides, I knew they were right. Hypoparathyroidism caused abnormal brain calcifications that could be seen on skull X-ray. Her skull X-rays had shown no such calcifications.

I had no idea what she had. Worse, I had no idea what to do.

I put her on a combination of levodopa plus bromocriptine and waited for some new insight or a new drug or both.

Six months later the first CAT scanner was installed in Chicago, the third in the United States. What excitement! To actually see the outline of the normal living brain. To see the images of the diseases themselves, brain tumors, hemorrhages, strokes, right there, before your own eyes.

In Parkinson's disease, the CAT scans were normal. The substantia nigra could not be seen, and its cell loss was too subtle a change for a CAT scan to pick up.

But I ordered one for Roberta.

"Why?" she asked me.

"Because I do not know what is wrong with your brain."

"Will knowing help me?"

"Of course," I replied blithely.

I ordered the CAT scan. It was done the next day. As soon as I finished rounds that day, I stopped by radiology to look at Roberta's scan.

One glance and I knew everything. Deep within each half of her brain, in the area of each striatum, there was a massive area of white. Calcium. Like two bricks deep inside the brain.

Roberta didn't have true Parkinson's disease. Such deposits of calcium deep in the brain are not part of Parkinson's disease.

Her Parkinsonism was due to a disorder of the striatum, of the cells that responded to dopamine, not of the cells of the substantia nigra that made dopamine. And I could see that disorder: Her striatum had been invaded by calcified tissue. That was why it could not respond to dopamine and so had the symptoms of parkinsonism. Parkinsonism with normal dopamine function, with normal HVA levels. Parkinsonism that did not respond to levodopa or bromocriptine or lergotrile.

And it was due to hypoparathyroidism from her thyroid surgery. That had to be what had caused her brain to become calcified.

I called her immediately.

She recognized the excitement in my voice. She listened hard to everything I said. And then she asked her same question.

"Will it help me?"

I started to shout my confident response, but stopped short. Her striatal tissue was calcified. Its dopamine receptors were damaged. Probably destroyed. We knew they would not respond to dopamine or bromocriptine or lergotrile. Our hope had been that some other drug, a cousin to bromocriptine, might work where bromocriptine had failed. One look back at the CAT scan shining out from the X-ray viewing box where I had left it made that possibility a pipe dream.

And treating her hypoparathyroidism might slow the progression of her disease, but it wouldn't dissolve those two bricks.

She repeated her question.

"Will it help me?"

I answered her as honestly as I could without giving up all hope. She understood all too well.

The endocrinologist proved that my diagnosis was correct and we treated her. It made no difference. Roberta Rose Richards slowly deteriorated. She died three years later.

Two years before she died, she became famous. I published her case history, replete with CAT scan, HVA levels, and failure of response to medications. She was the first pure instance in which a patient who looked and acted just like a patient with ordinary Parkinson's disease did not have Parkinson's disease. She had a Parkinsonlike disease due to a disorder of the striatum.

I worked very hard on that paper. It was of major theoretical importance in helping physicians and other scientists understand what is going on inside the brain in Parkinson's and related diseases.

Roberta in a way became noteworthy. The scientific world now understood that there were two separate ways of becoming parkinsonian—loss of dopamine producing cells and decrease of dopamine receiving cells (receptors). Roberta would have been far happier if the knowledge had helped her. And so would I.

Today, neurologists recognize the entity of levodopa-resistant Parkinsonlike disorders. I see about one such patient every couple of months. They all have something wrong in the striatum, and normal levels of HVA. There is still very little we can do to help most of them. Levodopa doesn't work, nor bromocriptine, nor its newer analogues. But for some, the outlook has changed. All such patients get CAT scans or MRI scans. And every once in a while these scans show calcification, which in some patients is due to hypoparathyroidism. I never see such a patient without thinking of Roberta Rose Richards and her recurring question, "Will it help me?" Now I have a better answer: If I see them early enough and treat their hypoparathyroidism. They don't get better, but at least they don't deteriorate the way Roberta did. I'm sure she'd have settled for that.

13

HUMAN EXPERIMENTATION

A drug is any substance which when given to a rat results in a paper.

Edgerton Y. Davis

Harvey Zeigler was the Lone Ranger. He was also Batman. And sometimes he was the Green Hornet, but not very often. There were even instances where he was all three at the same time. Only he was better. He was stronger, smarter, more cunning. And at those times he didn't need anyone to help him. He could do it all himself. He needed no Tonto. No Robin. No Cato. He didn't need any of them. He didn't miss them. They couldn't be trusted anyway. No one could be. He could defeat the Russians and their evil empire by himself. He'd stop them from taking over American TV.

They thought they were so smart. And they were. Far too clever for the FBI and the CIA, but not too clever for him. It was cable TV. That was their plan. Cable TV was not home entertainment. It was a way of putting a Russian agent in everyone's home. First to spy on everyone like Big Brother. He's read *1984*, and here it was, 1984, the real 1984. Why didn't the cops understand? Once the whole country was hooked up, then the cable TVs would do more than just spy. They'd take over. They'd give the orders and everyone would obey. A country of robots controlled by their own TV sets.

But they couldn't control him. They tried. He heard them. Voices from his TV set. Evil voices. Telling him to stop; telling him to help them. Help them! Never. He was a loyal American. He'd show them. He'd save the country. Thank God for telephone poles. He knew he could do what had to be done. And he'd be able to do it as long as he had his radio with him. And he could get the orders he needed from Captain Andy on the spaceship *Emily*. From Captain Andy to him. He was their only hope of saving America, of saving the earth. And he could do it as long as he had his radio and stayed within a hundred yards of a telephone pole. If he got any farther away, the signal wouldn't reach him. He had not had time to put in all that cable like the Russians had, so his messages came from the telephone poles. Thank God for AT&T.

And the government was breaking up AT&T. Didn't they know? Didn't they realize that America needed those monopolies to combat the Red Menace? If there were no telephone poles, then there would be no messages from Captain Andy. No signals from the spaceship *Emily*. And with no messages, there would be no Lone Ranger. No Batman. No Green Hornet. Just Harvey Zeigler with nothing he could do and no place to go. He couldn't go home. The Russians were there. Or into the corner bar. SportsVision. The Reds. Watching. Listening. Sending out their coded orders.

The Chicago police found Harvey at two in the morning walking around a telephone pole and talking into his radio. It was not talking back. The radio was not sending out any messages; it was emitting no sounds at all. It couldn't. It had no batteries. But that didn't stop Harvey. He kept right on talking to the radio. Talking and listening.

The police finally got his attention long enough to ask his name.

"The Lone Ranger," he replied. "Can't you tell from my mask?"

He wasn't wearing any mask.

"Where is Tonto?" one of the cops asked.

"The Russians killed him."

"How?"

"The usual way," he said knowingly.

"And how is that?"

"They poisoned the water."

"Then how come only Tonto died?"

"Others died too."

"Who?"

"Robin. Cato."

That was enough for them. They took the Lone Ranger to the Dearborn State Psychiatric Hospital. He clutched his radio during the entire trip. The hospital signed him in as Harvey Zeigler, having found his wallet in his pocket. He signed in as Bruce Wayne.

They made a diagnosis of acute paranoid schizophrenia. He needed treatment. Of that there was no doubt. But what treatment?

The Chief of Psychiatry at Dearborn State Psychiatric Hospital was doing research on a new antipsychotic drug. The resident who saw Harvey Zeigler, alias Bruce Wayne, thought he was a perfect candidate for this new medication. He fit the design of the study, the protocol, perfectly. He had the right diagnosis: acute paranoid schizophrenia. He was the right age, under forty. He had no other known diseases and he was not on any other antipsychotic medications. He was receiving no treatment at all. The ideal candidate. It was as if the study had been designed specifically for him.

The resident, Frank Hayes, asked him once again, "Have you seen any doctors recently?"

"No. They are all controlled by the Russians."

"They are?"

"Of course. Through their TVs. They all have TVs. Some even have them in their waiting rooms," he explained, still clutching his radio to his ear.

"I never watch TV," the resident said. "I don't even own one."

"You're smart. The Russians control the TVs. It's the cables." Harvey looked around. "Are there TVs here?"

"Not cable," the doctor assured him. "Just American TV."

Harvey put down his radio for the first time. He felt almost safe. This was someone he could trust.

Harvey was the perfect candidate. He was acutely crazy, paranoid as hell, and totally untreated. They had other options. They could give him any of the standard antipsychotics: Haldol, Thorazine, Prolixin. They would undoubtedly work. But such patients didn't come into the ER every night. He was ideal for TW-406. It would work. It would help him.

Dr. Hayes called his chief, Dr. Joseph Woods. He told Woods the whole story.

"He's a perfect candidate; enroll him. We need four more to complete the study. If we treat him, we'll only need three more. Get him signed up and started. I'll see him later."

Hayes hung up the phone.

"Who was that?" Harvey asked.

"Dr. Woods. He hates TV. Never watches it."

Harvey was skeptical.

"I've been to his house. He doesn't even own a TV set. He's going to help you."

"How?"

"He and I are going to give you a medicine that will help you combat the Russians."

"What medicine?"

"TW-406."

"I've never heard of that. What's its real name?"

135

"If I tell you, the Russians might find out. They're everywhere."

"That's right." Harvey looked around suspiciously. "TW-406," he whispered.

"But first you must sign this." With that explanation, Dr. Hayes handed Harvey a piece of paper entitled Consent Form.

"What's this?"

"A permission form."

"Permission for what?"

"To combat the Russians."

Harvey took the piece of paper and signed it. "Jay Silverheels."

Hayes knew that that was not his name. Why had he signed it that way?

To fool the Russians.

Jay Silverheels was given a plastic name tag with his correct name on it and was admitted to the acute ward. He was placed in a room without any TV set and after some blood was drawn for those routine blood tests that are required for any experimental medication, he was started on TW-406. TW-406 was an antipsychotic drug, a second cousin of haloperidol (Haldol), one of the standards of the field. Such drugs have revolutionized psychiatry. Before the introduction of such medications, patients like Harvey Zeigler, patients suffering through their first acute schizophrenic break with reality, stayed in places like Dearborn State for an average of about two years before they were organized enough to allow them to try to function on their own again. Today, that process takes an average of two to three weeks. Quite a difference. And dozens of such drugs are available. The first antipsychotic or neuroleptic, Thorazine, is still being used almost forty years after the serendipitous discovery that it calmed, soothed, and seemed to control schizophrenics. So are a couple of dozen other drugs with similar actions on the brain.

So why do we need another neuroleptic? Why TW-406? There are a number of answers, some medical or scientific, others not so scientific. The basic fact is that none of the neuroleptics cure schizophrenia. The process, whatever it is, goes on. The medication blunts and helps control the acute symptoms, the hallucinations, the delusions, the behaviors driven by such aberrant thought processes, but they do not cure the disease. They all work by inhibiting the activity of a specific chemical neurotransmitter called dopamine. This chemical, like other neurotransmitters, carries messages from one nerve cell to another, but not from all nerve cells nor to all other nerve cells. Only a few select group of cells, known as dopaminergic or dopamine-containing neurons, can produce and release dopamine. And not all nerve cells respond to dopamine. Only those neurons that contain highly specialized structures called dopamine receptors can receive messages from dopamine-producing neurons. It is these receptors that are the key to how antipsychotic drugs seem to work. These receptors respond to dopamine and their response determines the behavior of the neurons of which they are a part. As a result, the neuron can be inhibited or prevented from firing and thereby sending its message to other neurons, or it can be stimulated to send out its own neurotransmitters in search of other nerve cells and other receptors. And in some way, this process plays a role in producing behaviors, especially those peculiar behaviors that go to make up acute paranoid schizophrenia. Neuroleptics such as Thorazine and Haldol and all the others act by attaching to dopamine receptors and preventing dopamine from making contact with the receptor. This action of blocking dopamine receptors interrupts the transmission of messages and thereby inhibits those behaviors resulting from such transmissions.

But not all dopamine receptors are identical, so the exact pattern of dopamine-receptor blockade is different from neuroleptic to neuroleptic. That is the key to drug design. The perfect neuroleptic would only block those dopamine receptors involved in schizophrenia and would spare all others. Those others are involved in a wide variety of "normal" brain functions and their blockade results in a number of the side effects caused by these antipsychotic agents. These vary from sedation and confusion to drug-induced Parkinson-like states and abnormal involuntary movements. The perfect neuroleptic would only block the "right" receptors and would be devoid of all such unwanted side effects. Unfortunately, no such perfect neuroleptic has been discovered; the search for one is a very legitimate quest. It still would not cure schizophrenia. A cure would somehow end the process whereby dopamine produces abnormal behaviors. Neuroleptics do not end that process, they merely make it more difficult for dopamine to reach the receptor. Once neuroleptics are stopped, dopamine can again reach the receptor in an uninhibited fashion. As a result, about one of every ten schizophrenics who is taken off neuroleptics or who stops neuroleptics has an acute psychotic break within the first month, another 10 percent the second month, and so on, so that by six months half of the patients have had psychotic lapses.

That is one reason drug companies remain interested in developing new neuroleptics. There are a lot of schizophrenics in the world and, once placed on neuroleptics, they stay on them for years. The answer to a drug company's prayer. Hence TW-406. A new neuroleptic. A cousin of haloperidol. Developed with the hope that it would be different enough from haloperidol that it would have some advantage for at least some patients—less sedation, less parkinsonism, less nervousness, less of something—that would allow Williams Pharmaceuticals to get a share of the market. Not a big share, just a few percentages, say five hundred million dollars per year in sales worldwide.

So TW-406 was started. It worked, and within a few days Harvey was no longer clutching his radio to his ear. Within a week, he was no longer talking about the Russians. After two weeks he stopped mentioning the Lone Ranger, Batman, the Green Hornet, Captain Andy and Spaceship *Emily*. He started reading the newspapers each morning, starting with the sports page and rarely getting much farther, but according to his parents (who now were visiting him on a regular basis) that was fairly normal for him.

Dr. Hayes talked to the parents for some time. There was some background information he needed to be able to fill out on all the forms for TW-406. Was this the first time that Harvey had been hospitalized for a psychiatric disorder?

It was.

Perfect. That meant that this had been Harvey's first breakdown, his first attack of schizophrenia. All too often, patients came in and were put on a protocol for first-break schizophrenics only to be dropped from the study when it turned out that it was not their first episode. So far, so good.

Had he ever been treated with any antipsychotic drugs? Any neuroleptics? Any major tranquilizers?

No. No tranquilizers at all. As far as his parents knew, he'd never even seen a psychiatrist.

Wonderful. How long had he been sick? When had his behavior changed?

About six months earlier.

Their answers couldn't have been better. Harvey fit the protocol perfectly. It was as if the study had been designed precisely for him. Dr. Hayes thanked the Zeiglers and said goodbye. He never even mentioned the experimental protocol to them, or the fact that their son was on an experimental medication. Why should he? Harvey was an adult. He was over twenty-one. His medications were not his parents' business.

That night Harvey made another stop toward normality. He requested a TV so he could watch his Cubs play.

In due time, a TV was put in his room, but Harvey never turned it on. Instead, he started pacing to and fro. Back and forth across his room, from one wall to the other. His life became a succession of continuous movements. He never sat down for more than a few seconds at a time. He never stood still without moving his feet. Marching in place. He ate standing up, still marching.

The nurses noted the change immediately. So did Dr. Hayes. And also Dr. Woods, when he made his weekly rounds. "Akathisia," he remarked.

"Most likely," Hayes agreed. Akathisia is a well-known side effect of all neuroleptics. It probably has something to do with blocking one or more subsets of dopamine receptors. It happens with all neuroleptics, but some are more likely to cause it than others. This was the second time they'd seen it with TW-406. And they both recalled the other patient. They had decreased her daily dose of TW-406. The akathisia got worse. So did her psychosis. They doubled her dose. Her psychosis improved and so did the akathisia. In ten days the restlessness was gone. That rarely happened with other neuroleptics. Never with Haldol or Thorazine. Increasing the dose never improved true akathisia with most drugs. If it did with TW-406, that would be most exciting. It might be worth writing up for publication in a scientific journal since it might be a way of treating the often untreatable akathisia.

"I think we should increase his dose," Dr. Woods proposed.

"Just what I was thinking, Chief," Hayes concurred. "I'll double it." After all, that was what had worked before.

"Yes," Woods nodded, already walking off to the next room.

Within two days, Harvey was able to sit through lunch without once moving his feet and then sat still through an entire Cubs game, a 7–0 loss to San Diego.

That night Harvey ran a low-grade fever—100.6. No big deal. He had no other symptoms except a mild stiffness of his arms and legs. The next morning, he was even stiffer and much quieter than usual. He didn't talk about the ballgame at all. He didn't read the sports section. He just sat in a chair and stared at the wall, hardly moving a muscle.

Harvey also skipped lunch. He still had a low-grade fever. The nurses called Hayes. He took a look at Harvey. Harvey was mute, immobile. Hayes tried to get him talk about the Cubs but got no response.

The Russians.

Nothing.

The Lone Ranger.

Zip.

Batman. The Green Hornet.

A blank stare.

Captain Andy.

A smile. Faint, but a smile nonetheless.

Hayes was disappointed. He was certain that the medication was not doing its job. Harvey had obviously withdrawn from reality. He was back to his fantasy world, living with his delusions. And that world had once again taken over from the real world. Harvey had gotten worse.

What to do? Should he switch him to another neuroleptic and give up on the TW-406? No. It was too soon to give up. He'd increase the dose. They had started at 200 milligrams per day. Harvey was now on 400 milligrams per day. The protocol allowed for up to 800; 800 he would get.

And he did.

That night Harvey's temperature went up to 105. His body became so stiff that the nurses could hardly bend his arms.

That was how I first heard about Harvey Zeigler. Hayes called Woods. Woods told him to call me. He did and he told me about the patient. He described him as a patient with viral encephalitis. That was their diagnosis.

"What virus?" I asked.

"Herpes encephalitis," I was told. Herpes encephalitis is caused by the herpes simplex virus. This type of virus causes canker sores. It is the commonest of all viral encephalitis but, more significant, it is also the one viral encephalitis that commonly starts by causing a change in behavior that is initially interpreted as a psychosis. About once a year I'd get a call from a resident at Dearborn State about a patient with encephalitis. The story was always the same. A change of behavior. Psychiatric admission. Treatment. Coma with seizures. Fever. All within two to three weeks.

The details varied from patient to patient. Some had been paranoid, some withdrawn, some confused. The exact nature of the psychiatric histories were so variable that they hardly mattered. I only half-listened as Hayes went on and on about the Lone Ranger and the

Russians. It was like listening to the world's longest shaggy-dog story, hoping that the punch line would be good enough to make it all worthwhile and redeem the effort of listening.

He got to the end. There was no real punch line. No redemption. And no seizures.

Sometimes that happened in herpes encephalitis. One slightly atypical feature. "How long has he been in Dearborn?" I asked.

"Five weeks," he told me.

"Herpes doesn't go on for five weeks and then explode like this. Either the patients go to hell in a couple of weeks or they get better."

"He got better for a while."

"That doesn't happen, either," I replied.

"It doesn't?"

"How long had he been psychotic?" I asked.

"Six months."

"It's not herpes. That never drags on for six months. It's an acute infection, not a chronic illness."

"So what's he got?" Hayes asked.

"Tell me the story again," I suggested.

He did. And this time I listened as carefully as I could. And he told it as carefully as he could. A far different scenario emerged. The patient had gone through a period of at least six months of progressive psychosis. Plain, old-fashioned paranoid schizophrenia. He then received treatment with a neuroleptic. That was standard procedure and was followed by clinically obvious improvement, as often occurred. This was then followed by the emergence of side effects. Nothing at all unusual about that. He was given a larger dose and got worse. More side effects. Fever. Stiffness.

More neuroleptic.

Disaster. High fever. A change in his behavior. Severe rigidity.

"Neuroleptic malignant syndrome," I said.

"Are you sure?"

"Pretty sure."

"But I've never seen it with TW-406."

"It happens only in one of a thousand patients or so. How many people have you treated with that drug?"

"Fifteen."

"I rest my case."

"Are you sure TW-406 can cause neuroleptic malignant syndrome?"

"Yes."

141

"How can you be so sure?"
"It's a neuroleptic. They all do."

Two hours later Harvey Zeigler arrived at our hospital, transferred by ambulance. Within another three hours we were certain of the diagnosis. Neuroleptic malignant syndrome is a clinical diagnosis. That phrase means that the diagnosis is based primarily on clinical judgment. There is no test that proves whether or not the patient has neuroleptic malignant syndrome. Good clinical judgment is made up of two sets of information. The first is the clinical picture presented by the patient. Is the clinical picture consistent with the diagnosis? In order to answer this question, the clinician must know the basic components of the disease and all of its variations and ramifications.

Neuroleptic malignant syndrome was first described in the mid-1950s, shortly after the initial widespread use of the original neuroleptics. By the 1980s, the components of this syndrome were well known. Everyone who used neuroleptics regularly knew that it could happen. The problem only occurs, of course, in patients receiving neuroleptics. While neuroleptic malignant syndrome can strike at almost any time, it usually appears soon after the patient is started on the drug, or within a week or two following an increase in the daily dose. Three things happen to the patient. The first is a fever. The patient, for no apparent reason, begins to run a temperature. There is no other evidence of an infection and, most of the time, no infection exists. At first, the temperature is often rather low, but then it quickly jumps to alarming levels, the kind of level only rarely seen in adults—105 degrees, 106 degrees, even higher.

Despite these extreme temperatures, there is still no sign of infection and no infection. If there is no infection, where does the fever come from? It comes from the brain, from that small area in the brain in the hypothalamus where body temperature is regulated. This temperature-regulating center is made up of nerve cells, nerve cells with a variety of receptors including dopamine receptors. These are not the dopamine receptors involved in schizophrenia, but they are dopamine receptors and they can be blocked by neuroleptics. And that blockade can, at times, result in a dramatic change in function, like an unexplained fever of 105 or more.

Harvey Zeigler's fever was 106.8 degrees when he arrived at our hospital.

The second component is severe stiffness in which the muscles become very rigid, almost in a state of rigor mortis. The patient's arms and legs may be extended straight out or the patient may be bent into a fetal posture; any combination can occur. But whatever the posture, the key element is always the same, moving the arms or a leg or the neck is like trying to bend a lead pipe.

Harvey's arms were bent across his chest like the arms of an ancient Egyptian mummy. His legs were straight with his feet pointing down. His head was bent forward and nothing could be moved. Lead-pipe rigidity.

How does this happen? The neuroleptic had blocked the dopamine receptors of the motor system, the ones related to control of movement, and now all of those cells were maximally excited and firing like mad. And there was Harvey, a burning mummy.

This type of extreme posture involves massive work on the part of the muscles, as a result of which the muscles release an enzyme, creatinine phosphokinase (known as CPK) into the blood. The level of this enzyme is always increased in neuroleptic malignant syndrome. It is the one laboratory test that is positive. In our lab, the upper limit of normal is sixty. Harvey's level was above three thousand.

The last component of the triad consists of changes in behavior. These often begin rather subtly as simple agitation or confusion but often progress into states of stupor or coma.

Harvey was stuporous. Only the most vigorous stimulation could wake him up, and even when aroused he was confused. It was 1977. He was in Gotham City. But he knew his name: Harvey Zeigler.

Harvey manifested all of the right signs and symptoms:

Fever 106.8°.

Severe rigidity.

Stupor and confusion.

His CPK was markedly elevated. The diagnosis was staring us in the face.

But could he have anything else? Was there any other cause for his fever? Did he have an infection? This is the second step in making a clinical diagnosis—ruling out other significant diseases the patient could have, especially any treatable illnesses.

His white blood count was normal, as were all his other blood tests. All except the elevated CPK. We did a spinal tap and examined his spinal fluid for any possible signs of infection; we found none. We performed a CAT scan to rule out an abscess in the brain, the scan was normal. We were done. We had ruled out all other possible diagnoses. We were left just where we'd started.

Neuroleptic malignant syndrome.

We knew the diagnosis and could make a good guess as to the prognosis. That was not as good as we'd have liked. Although most patients with neuroleptic malignant syndrome make a good recovery, too many such patients have died. Others have been left with severe neurologic damage. What could we do to help Harvey? First, we had to make sure nothing went wrong. We put in an IV to keep him hydrated and give his muscles and body needed nourishment. We monitored his heart. Sudden changes in his heart rhythm could be fatal. We put him on a respirator and controlled his respiration, making certain that he got sufficient oxygen to his brain and liver and kidneys.

All of that was well and good. We were preventing complications, but was there anything we could actually do to help him more positively? There was no proven treatment, but other physicians had reported positive results with a variety of approaches. Some used muscle relaxants devised to treat muscle rigidity seen in MS or strokes. Some used anti-Parkinson agents. These reduced the rigidity of Parkinson's disease by acting at the dopamine receptors. These are the same receptors the neuroleptics attacked. It was hoped that these drugs might reduce the stiffness.

We gave Harvey both types of medication. Within twelve hours his muscles began to relax. We could move his arms and legs. It took a lot of effort, but we could move them. His temperature came down to 103. He was easier to arouse and less confused. He was far from cured, but the crisis had passed. He was no longer a mummy whose body was burning up before our eyes. He would survive.

It took another week before the last elements of Harvey's neuroleptic malignant syndrome cleared. No more fever, no more stupor, no more confusion. He knew who he was, where he was, what the date was, why he was in the hospital, who we all were. He was back to normal, back to his old self. His schizophrenia was in remission. He still distrusted the government, but who doesn't from time to time?

His muscles did not go back to normal. His arms were still bent part way across his chest. His fists were clenched. His legs stuck out straight with his feet pointed down. He could hardly bend his elbows or his wrists or his knees or his hips, and he could not move his hands or feet. Nor could we. He had developed contractures—fixed postures due to brain and muscle injury—a permanent residue of his neuroleptic malignant syndrome.

Harvey went from our hospital to a rehabilitation center for extensive physical therapy. After he was discharged, I sent a copy of his discharge summary to the referring physician, Dr. Joseph Woods. I always do that. The final diagnosis was Neuroleptic Malignant Syndrome due to TW-406. I also called Woods to tell him about it. After all, TW-406 was an experimental drug. He was the chief investigator. He was obligated to report any and all serious complications to the manufacturers and to the FDA. He didn't seem too pleased by the call. It was almost as if I were attacking him and the drug. I wasn't. I was just keeping him informed.

He thanked me.

Over the next year, I saw Harvey twice. He made significant progress, but despite prolonged rehabilitation, he still had severe problems. He had required surgical procedures to get his feet into a position so that he could walk. Not normally, but with a slow shuffling gait. He could move his hands but awkwardly, clumsily. He could hardly write his name. Each time I saw him, I dictated a note and sent it to Joseph Woods. It was information he needed, that the manufacturers needed, and that the FDA needed.

Then Harvey Zeigler disappeared from my practice but not my life. A lawyer I'd never heard of named Roger Merzbacker subpoenaed my records. Harvey was suing Joseph Woods, Frank Hayes, and Williams Pharmaceuticals. I was, in legal parlance, a "subsequent treating physician." I had to respond to the subpoena and had to act as a witness to the various medical facts of the patient's illness if so asked. I was and in due time my deposition was scheduled.

In such a lawsuit, the plaintiff must prove several things. Each must be shown to have occurred "more probably than not," for that is the burden of proof in a civil suit.

What did Roger Merzbacker have to prove more probably than not? The usual triad, deviation, causation, permanence. He had to show that the defendants had been negligent, that they had done something they should not have done, something that was a deviation from the standard of care. Then they had to show that this deviation was the cause of some sort of damage and that the damage was permanent. Invariably this is done through the testimony of expert witnesses, with the experts of one side saying one thing and those on the other side saying something else. In my deposition I would not be a hired expert. I would be a subsequent treating physician. As such, I could not be forced to give opinions; all I would have to testify to were the facts, but often a jury gives more weight to what a treating physician has to say than to experts called in after the facts. I would be a key witness and the facts I would testify to would be two-thirds of the case. Causation and permanence.

The deposition took place in the conference room of one of the large law firms in downtown Chicago. At nine-thirty I walked into a room full of lawyers. Roger Merzbacker was there representing Harvey Zeigler. And there were a host of other lawyers representing the various defendants. Three were representing Williams Pharmaceuticals. They were accompanied by the director of Clinical Pharmacology. One represented Joseph Woods, one Frank Hayes, one the nurses at Dearborn, and two the hospital itself.

Why all the lawyers? What were the issues? I had no idea. Harvey had had neuroleptic malignant syndrome. It was a known complication of all neuroleptics. Its occurrence did not imply malpractice.

The deposition began. Depositions of subsequent treating physicians are usually fairly benign affairs. Such physicians are assumed to be neutral and their neutrality is respected. The last thing anyone wants to do is to annoy a neutral party and transform him into an advocate for the other side.

Did I know Harvey Zeigler?

I did. He was my patient.

How had he become my patient?

I told them the story.

Had I made a diagnosis?

I had.

What was that diagnosis?

"Neuroleptic Malignant Syndrome due to TW-406."

Merzbacker asked me to explain Neuroleptic Malignant Syndrome and I did.

He asked me how I'd made the diagnosis and I told him.

Was I sure of my diagnosis?

I was.

"Are you sure within a reasonable degree of medical certainty that Mr. Zeigler had neuroleptic malignant syndrome?"

I recognized the formulation. This was the key question framed as it would be for an expert.

"Yes," I replied. "There is no doubt in my mind that Harvey had neuroleptic malignant syndrome."

"Do you have an opinion as to what caused his neuroleptic

malignant syndrome?"

"Yes."

"And what is that opinion?"

"It was caused by TW-406."

"Do you hold that opinion to a reasonable degree of medical certainty?"

Back to the formula. "Yes."

They had causation. Merzbacker went on the next issue, permanence.

When had I last seen Mr. Zeigler? What were the findings? His disabilities? Would he get any better?

I answered. He was severely disabled and always would be. Merzbacker had permanence.

Did I have any other opinions?

"No."

I got up to leave.

"I have a couple of questions," one of the other lawyers said. His name was Kevin O'Rourke. He was one of the lawyers who represented the manufacturers of TW-406.

How long had I known about neuroleptic malignant syndrome? Years.

Was it a known problem with neuroleptics?

It was.

With all neuroleptics?

Yes.

Would a manufacturer be negligent for making a neuroleptic that caused neuroleptic malignant syndrome?

Of course not.

Why not?

"They all cause neuroleptic malignant syndrome."

"All neuroleptics?"

"Yes."

He smiled. He's made his point. Merzbacker might have causation and permanence, but he didn't have negligence, not on the part of Williams Pharmaceuticals. No negligence. No deviation. No case.

The ball was back in Merzbacker's court.

"Neuroleptic malignant syndrome is a known complication of all neuroleptics," he began.

I agreed.

Should Williams Pharmaceuticals have known that?

Of course.

And Dr. Woods?

Yes.

And Dr. Hayes?

Yes.

Should Mr. Zeigler have been warned, since this was an experimental drug?

He got the question out so quickly and I answered so quickly that no one had time to object.

"Yes," I said.

Was he?

They all objected.

I had no idea what Merzbacker was driving at.

Merzbacker handed me the consent form for the TW-406. In describing the drug, it referred to TW-406 as safe and like all other neuroleptics free of serious side effects.

Did I agree with that statement?

Objections galore.

"No," I replied. In a deposition all objections are recorded and then the question is answered since there is no judge present to act on the objections.

"Was the consent form adequate?"

"No."

"Do you have opinion as to whether the consent form's failure to mention the possibility of serious side effects was a deviation from the standard of care?"

More objections. What made me an expert on informed consent?

Fifteen years of clinical research. Fifteen years as a consultant to drug companies.

More objections. Arguments. Side issues.

My answer. "Yes. It was a deviation." Deviation. The third element.

On whose part?

Everyone's. The manufacturer which approved the form. The hospital committee which approved the form. Dr. Woods as chief investigator.

Anyone else?

No.

Dr. Hayes?

No. He had nothing to do with drawing up the form.

Hayes' lawyer was relieved.

The nurse who was the witness? Did she have any control over the content of the form?

No.

Another happy lawyer.

"So neither Hayes nor the nurse was negligent," Hayes' lawyer said, ready to walk out scot-free.

"No. They were both as guilty as hell," I said.

The room was suddenly as quiet as it could get.

"Look at the signature. Jay Silverheels. Zeigler was, as we say in the medical trade, as nutty as a loon. This consent form is meaningless. And Hayes obtained that signature and the nurse witnessed it."

We all went around the same issues for another two hours, but the case was over. In the next few months everyone settled. Harvey Zeigler is said to have received about a million and a half dollars. It is rumored that when the antique auto museum in Highland Park auctioned off all its cars, Harvey bought the original TV Batmobile. That was before the movie *Batman* was made.

But the case was not over for me. I'm not sure it ever will be. I don't see Harvey Zeigler as a patient. Dearborn State no longer refers any of their patients to me. Joseph Woods walks by me at medical meetings without even nodding his head to acknowledge my presence. And Williams Pharmaceuticals refused to allow me to study a new anti-Parkinson drug they tried to develop. TW-406 it turns out, was not a very good neuroleptic. They stopped studying it about the time of my deposition in 1982.

Four years after the case was settled, Rush University, where I have been since 1977, was looking for someone to become Chairman of Neurology. I was a candidate. Or least I thought so until I talked to the dean.

He did not think I'd make a good chairman.

Why not? My research?

No. He respected my research. I'd published more scientific papers than any neurologist he knew.

My teaching?

No. I had won the teaching award, voted on by the medical students. No problem there.

My administrative skills?

No.

My clinical skills? My ability to attract patients?

No.

Then why? After all, these were the aspects of the job description of a chairman. Research, teaching, administration, and patient care. What else was there?

"Why?" I asked.

"You testify against physicians. And hospitals."

"Never."

"Mr. Zeigler."

"He was my patient. I testified for him. Not against anybody."

"You testified against Dearborn State," the dean told me.

"But didn't he deserve his day in court?"

"That cost us patient referrals."

And that was that. Hospitals are big businesses. They focus on the bottom line. Perhaps they have to. It's a tough world. But the world was also tough for Harvey Zeigler, and what happened to him at Dearborn State made it tougher. His million plus dollars didn't make him whole again. No amount of money could do that. Not even the Batmobile could do that.

14

No Harm, No Foul

It is one thing to show a man that he is in error, and another to put him in possession of the truth.

John Locke

It seems that no week goes by without some lawyer I do not know calling my office to ask me if I would be willing to be an expert witness in a case. Usually I have no idea how any of these lawyers have gotten my name. I am not listed with any service that supplies expert witnesses; nonetheless, lawyers find me. Joan McAnany was an exception. She found my name in the *Index Medicus*, a monthly compendium of scientific publications in medicine and related scientific fields. She worked for a legal defense firm that had been hired to defend a pharmaceutical company, Sterling Drugs, in a lawsuit. Sterling Drugs manufactured a dye used in myelograms known as Amipaque or metrizamide. The suit alleged that the Amipaque had resulted in brain damage in a patient who had undergone a metrizamide (Amipaque) myelogram. So Joan McAnany had gone to the library and looked up metrizamide in the *Index Medicus* and out popped my name. I had been the senior co-author of a publication which reviewed all of the neurologic complications of metrizamide. To her, that made me just the expert she wanted, so she called me. She asked me if I was willing to be an expert witness for her client.

I told her that I would be happy to review the records and tell her my thoughts about the case. Then, if what I thought coincided with what she and her clients wanted to present in court, I'd probably be willing to be an expert witness.

That was what she'd meant.

I had become an expert on metrizamide almost by accident. I had not planned to write that article. It was not an area of neurology, or neuropharmacology for that matter, in which I had any particular interest. But I have always had an overriding interest in the academic development of my residents. One of the major obstacles in their academic growth is writing that first major paper. Aron Buchman was one of my residents and wanted to pursue an academic career. During his training he'd taken care of two or three patients who had developed neurologic problems following myelograms performed using metrizamide. He started reading the entire medical literature on the subject. There wasn't that much, and there wasn't a single good review article putting all of the scattered information together. He wanted to write one, but he needed a senior investigator to help him; someone with a known level of expertise in pharmacology to judge, criticize, and direct his work. Someone like me. Would I help him?

Of course. So we went to work. And in due time, I became a recognized authority on the neurologic complications of metrizamide, a published authority. Metrizamide can and does cause neurologic problems, but it is a reasonably safe drug. Far safer than the older drugs that it replaced. Its development was a significant step forward in the efforts to produce a totally safe, "ideal" contrast agent for such studies. Unfortunately, that goal had not yet been reached.

I received the records from Joan McAnany two days later. I also received a copy of the plaintiff's deposition and the depositions of several of the defendants. Overall, it was more material than I really wanted to read.

The plaintiff's name was Rivera, Louis Rivera. His lawyer's name was William Goodman. Rivera was twenty-four years old. He'd gone to see a Dr. Phillip Landis. Rivera had hurt his back at work. He worked delivering newspapers. He hurt himself throwing newspapers off the truck. The pain stayed mostly in his back, but sometimes it shot down his right leg.

Two weeks off work didn't help.

Muscle relaxants didn't help.

Nor did anything else.

Dr. Landis was an orthopedic surgeon. He ordered an EMG. It didn't show much. Landis felt that Rivera needed to have a myelogram to see if an operation was necessary.

An operation for what, Rivera asked him.

A ruptured disc.

Would the operation help?

If he had a ruptured disc.

Rivera went into the hospital. A radiologist there did the myelogram; his name was Romano. Rivera didn't even remember meeting him. He remembered the myelogram though, every painful moment of it. And the headache it caused. And ever since then, he had trouble thinking. He couldn't concentrate. His memory was shot. He couldn't remember anything.

He told Dr. Landis about his headaches.

Dr. Landis blamed the metrizamide. And said the headaches would get better. They did, but nothing else did.

So Rivera got himself a lawyer, a guy named Phillips. Phillips was a general attorney. He referred Rivera to Goodman. Goodman specialized in malpractice. Goodman filed the suit. He sued everybody in sight. Sterling Drugs. Landis. Romano. The hospital.

Now he had to build his case. To do that, he needed to prove four separate elements. The first was negligence. For the physicians, that meant that it would have to be shown that they had either done something they should not have done or not done something they should have done—sins of commission or sins of omission. Either would do. For Sterling Drugs, it had to be shown that either they made an unsafe drug or failed to warn the users of any possible damage. Then he had to prove that his client was injured (damages), hopefully permanently (permanence). And then he had to put it altogether and prove that the negligence caused the permanent injury (causation).

Goodman started by sending his client to see a psychologist. If there were no damages, what difference would negligence make?

The psychologist tested him. Rivera's IQ was 81, below normal. Just what they needed. Proof that Rivera had suffered damage. Brain damage.

The psychologist tested Rivera again six months later. The second time his IQ was 79. He certainly was not getting better. The second element of their case was now in place. They had permanence.

All they needed now was causation.

And that they already had. Dr. Landis had said it was the metrizamide. Metrizamide could cause brain damage. He had told Rivera that, and he had repeated that statement in his deposition.

How did he know that?

He had read an article by somebody named Buchman. My article!

Romano agreed. He'd read the same article.

So much for my review.

Most of the case was in place. Causation, damages, permanence. And Sterling Drugs made that unsafe drug and no one warned the patient that such a terrible thing could result from such a simple procedure.

I called McAnany.

"Can we defend it?" she asked. "They want two million dollars. We offered one hundred thousand to make them go away. They turned us down."

"I don't believe their case," I said.

"Why not?"

"Metrizamide is pretty much like most other chemicals. If it causes a toxic reaction, that reaction is the worst when the concentration is highest. At the time of the myelogram Rivera had no problem. None at all, no convulsion, no seizure, no coma. No changes at all. Nothing. He remembers the entire procedure. He got a headache the next day. Everybody gets that from a myelogram. It's no big deal."

"So?"

"So, there is not a single patient in the medical literature with significant brain injury from metrizamide who didn't have a problem at the time of the myelogram."

"Are you sure of that?"

"I'm the expert," I reminded her.

"So what do we do?"

"Prove there was no damage."

"How do we do that?"

"Get his educational records. We'll see if he ever got tested before."

The records arrived four weeks later. Rivera was a high school dropout. He'd quit at age seventeen after finishing only three semesters. He was well over two years behind at that time. In a class of 827 he ranked below 750. Below that, the school didn't attempt an exact ranking. There seemed to be no purpose in it. College admission was not an issue.

That was all I needed.

I called McAnany.

"No harm, no foul," I said.

She didn't understand.

"Like the NBA," I explained.

That didn't help.

"Professional basketball. In the last minute of a game, the referees let the players play the game. They don't call fouls unless the players really get hurt. No harm—no foul."

She still wasn't following me.

"Rivera," I said, "is no stupider now than he ever was."

That she understood.

A month later, the lawyers all came up to Chicago for my deposition. I expressed my opinion in the proper legal terms. More probably than not, Mr. Rivera had not suffered any damage from metrizamide.

Goodman demanded to know the basis of my opinions.

There was no evidence of any acute neurologic problem at the time of his exposure to metrizamide and there was no evidence at all from the literature that metrizamide could cause permanent neurologic damage in the absence of any acute effect. Besides, there was no evidence of any damage.

None? William Goodman challenged me on that assertion. He asked me about Rivera's two IQ evaluations of 81 and 79.

I was ready for that question. I told him that in my opinion, more probably than not, his IQ was no different than it had ever been. The average IQ of dropouts from the lowest 10 percent of a high school class is no higher than 80.

No harm, no foul.

Soon afterward, Goodman offered to settle the case. After all, the witnesses to causation had all depended on one authority—me. And his proof of damages was shaky, to say the least.

He'd told McAnany that he'd take the hundred grand.

She offered twenty-five. That was less money than a trial would cost.

Goodman took the money.

LIVE CELLS FROM DEAD BABIES

A desperate disease requires a dangerous remedy.

Guy Fawkes

There is nothing more productive of problems than a really good solution.

Nathan S. Kline, MD

"Why," she asked, "must you use cells from a dead baby?"

I took a deep breath before I answered her. As far as I knew, Mrs. Romney was not an angry fanatic who equated abortion with murder and fetal research with the type of war crimes that Mengele had committed. Those critics cannot be answered. It is faith, not science, that sways them. She was the wife of one of my patients who had Parkinson's disease. I had been treating her husband for almost a decade. I met her on the initial visit but then did not see her again until his disability progressed to the point where he had trouble getting to the office by himself. Three or four years previously she had started accompanying him for some of the visits. Over the last two years, she'd brought him to each appointment. Mrs. Romney wanted to understand why fetal-cell studies were important for her and her husband. Why should she support such research? Deep down in her heart she didn't really approve of abortions.

It was, I reminded myself, best to begin at the beginning. Patients and their wives often get newsletters on Parkinson's disease. The various Parkinson's disease–oriented charities do what they can to help educate patients and their families. Patients and caregivers frequently study such information and they also ask me questions at every opportunity. Still, they aren't medical students. They neither remember nor understand the flurry of facts they are exposed to.

They do not have the kind of background that makes that easy. So I began at the very beginning, basic neuroscience. Neurology for the patient. "Brain cells are in many ways the most specialized cells of the body. Each of these nerve cells receive a series of inputs from other neurons and then relays a specific message to still other cells. The development of these special capabilities is associated with the loss of one major property almost all other adult cells in the human body have. Neurons cannot reproduce themselves. Other cells can. Liver cells, skin cells, lung cells, blood cells, bone cells, but not brain cells. Once a neuron dies, the brain has one less neuron. Other neurons cannot divide to replace that missing cell. Dead is dead. Gone.

"Now in a healthy brain," I continued, "that doesn't make much difference; we have more cells than we need. But in a diseased brain, that's not true. In Parkinson's disease, a specific group of neurons die, a group of cells known as the substantia nigra. It is the death of these cells and the lack of the messages they normally transmit that causes Parkinson's disease."

"What kills the cells?" she asked.

"That we don't know," I admitted, "and since we don't know, there's nothing we can do to prevent more cells from dying and the disease from progressing. There are several theories." I reminded her about Vitamin E. A number of research workers thought that Vitamin E by blocking excessive oxidation might slow down the rate of nerve cell death in Parkinson's disease. Mr. Romney was already taking Vitamin E. I also told her about the research that was going on with deprenyl, which was also thought to slow down the rate of nerve cell death. We and others were doing research to see if this might be true.

"And," she added, "my husband is taking medicine for his Parkinson's disease, Sinemet and Parlodel."

"Those medicines replace the chemical the substantia nigra makes, a chemical called dopamine, but the cells continue to die off and as they do, the substitutes become less and less effective."

"I know," she said softly. "He did so well for so many years . . . ." Her voice trailed off.

"There may be some other things we can try." I was as reassuring as I could be without painting a false picture.

"But why cells from babies?"

Back to the same question. Why couldn't we use substantia nigra cells from people who had been born and lived and then died? Then there would be no moral issue for her. It would be the same as heart transplants and liver transplants. But dead babies. Abortions.

That was totally different.

"But we can't do that. We can take a heart from someone who died in an accident and use, it but not part of the brain."

"Why not?"

"Because in order to take the heart, the brain must already be dead. That's how you determine that the heart donor is dead. It's called brain death. The heart is alive and healthy. It can be used. So can the liver, the kidneys, the cornea. But not the brain. And for the brain to be dead, the brain cells must all be dead. And for brain cells, dead is dead," I reiterated.

She nodded. "But does it have to be poor little fetuses?"

She hadn't said babies this time; perhaps that showed some progress. "Couldn't you take the cells out of someone dying of a brain tumor who needed brain surgery?"

"We couldn't. A brain cell is like a tree. Each cell of the substantia nigra sends out a single trunk which then branches out to reach thousands upon thousands of other cells. In an adult, taking out the cell body would be like sawing off a tree at ground level. The stump would die."

"And dead is dead," she said.

"Yes," I agreed, "but in a young fetus the trunk has not formed yet so we can take the entire tree and put it into the brain. There the cells would live and reproduce and form their trunks."

"Will that cure my husband?"

"I have no idea, but, unless we can do the research, we'll never know."

I thought that our conversation was over, that we could now move on to talking about her husband. I was wrong. She had one further question. "Who gives the permission?"

"Which permission?"

"To use the baby's tissue."

"The mo—" I stopped myself. She had gone back to *baby*. I would not go back to *mother*. Some issues go very deep. "The woman."

"But she just agreed to . . . ." This time she stopped herself. "I was going to say, 'kill her baby.'"

"I know. Once you say that, you've closed the door. The mother"—I chose that word carefully—"is a murderer. She can't give permission to use tissue from her murdered child. And if you work with her, you are no more than accessory to murder. Doing illegal experiments. Some Nazi war criminal."

159

She nodded.

"But abortion is only murder to some people. Not to all people. And it's not illegal. There are some safeguards to follow. We should never be out soliciting abortions. Never. But if a woman is going to have one, then why just destroy the fetus? Science can put it to good use."

"My husband," she began. The discussion was over. She wanted to get back to the day-to-day problem of trying to help her husband get out of bed by himself at night so that he could go to the bathroom with some semblance of dignity.

This conversation took place in early 1988. Fetal implants were all the rage then, both scientifically and politically. Such implants definitely helped animals with Parkinsonlike states. Would they help patients? Initial studies were being done. In Sweden. In China. In Cuba. In England. In Mexico. Even in the United States. Then the government banned the use of federal money to support such studies in the United States. It was an executive decision, made by the Reagan administration, a decision that controlled the National Institutes of Health purse strings. The NIH appointed a panel to advise them. I testified before that panel, representing several of the Parkinson's disease organizations. The panel heard all the evidence and voted unanimously. The NIH should expand its support of fetal research. Not just for Parkinsons, but in other diseases too, such as diabetes.

The Reagan administration did not lift the ban, nor has the Bush administration.

Politics at work.

Whether or not such implants will become an acceptable treatment in Parkinson's disease remains unproved, but it is a scientific question—not a political one. And like all scientific issues it has moral and ethical aspects. Ethical issues used to be considered by clinicians; today we have ethicists of medicine who have never taken care of sick people.

My first encounter with an ethicist was not a success. We hosted a minisymposium on brain implants as part of University Week at our University, and the organizers of the program felt that we should have someone speak on the ethics of fetal implantation. I was skeptical. To me, there was no ethical issue. Abortion was legal. The fetus is dead. All brain implants use brain cells from nonviable and therefore dead fetuses. The body belongs to the next of kin, who has the legal right to donate that body for legitimate research purposes.

But others had different points of view, and besides, the ethicist was going to be on campus that week and wouldn't cost us very much and the Office of Research would pay the honorarium.

For free, take.

We agreed.

The ethicist made her presentation and outlined a rather comprehensive set of ethical rules:

1. There should be no mention of donation until the woman has decided for other reasons to have an abortion. That is, no effort at coercing the woman to have an abortion.
2. There should be no relation between the woman/fetus and the recipient. No one should become pregnant just to supply needed fetal tissue to a relative or friend.
3. The fetus must be nonviable.
4. No one should make a profit from fetal tissue.

There were other similar guidelines. All equally benign and logical. But there was also an *or*. An ethical *or*. These rules could all be ignored if the government legally approved of any other alternative process.

"Which government?" someone asked her. At the time, the only implants had been done in Mexico and Sweden and the only one that had been proclaimed publicly had been in Mexico.

"The government of the country involved," she replied.

"So whatever the Mexican government says, the surgeon can do, and it's ethical," I said. "After all, Mexico has long been a model of ethical behavior."

"Yes," she agreed vigorously, seeing that I understood.

"And this government for us."

"Yes," she nodded vigorously.

"And the Third Reich for Mengele," I concluded, turning to leave as she sputtered.

I recalled the scene from Mel Brooks' classic *History of the World, Part I.* The scene took place just outside the Roman Senate. A Roman was in line at the unemployment office:

"What do you do for a living?" the clerk asked.

"I'm a stand-up philosopher."

"A bullshitter. Well, did you bullshit today?"

"No."

"Did you try to bullshit today?"

16

MY MOTHER'S AXIOM

God is trying to blow out the candle and I'm quickly trying to shield the flame taking advantage of His brief inattention.

> Marek Edelman, MD
> Cardiovascular Surgeon;
> The last surviving leader
> of the Warsaw ghetto uprising

There are, so the saying goes, no atheists in foxholes. I do not know whether that is true or not; I'm not sure anyone does. Has a survey ever been taken and the data collected, and is it accurate? Or are there "false positives," individuals who in that circumstance will claim to believe in God when in reality they do not? Who knows? The saying has been repeated so often it has become an axiom.

My mother had her own axiom. No antivivisectionist ever refused a life-saving Cesarean section because the technique had been perfected on dogs. Or because the obstetrician had himself perfected his own skills working on some animal other than humans. Did my mother have such data? Had she taken a survey? It was, I remind you, an axiom.

People, I suppose, have a right to oppose experimentation on animals. No scientific basis, but a right. And they have a right to oppose fetal implants. Not to equate it with Nazi war crimes. Not to declare it immoral or unethical or illegal until such time, if ever, the laws are changed. That will still not change the morals.

But they have their rights.

And with those rights there should come some obligations.

If medical research on animals is to be banned, a substitute must be found. One suggestion, for much of the needed work—human volunteers for those questions which can only be answered in that way. And all antivivisectionists owe it to the rest of society to volunteer. The line forms here. My mother's axiom: There are no antivivisectionists in that line.

If fetuses cannot be used, medical science will need more organ donors. Many more. And it's easy to sign up.

Is there a clamor of volunteers?

Or another axiom?

17

ONE STEP AHEAD

There must have been a moment, at the beginning, where we could have said—No.

Tom Stoppard
Rosencrantz and Guildenstern Are Dead

We are what we pretend to be so we must be careful about what we pretend to be.

Kurt Vonnegut
Mother Night

Alexa Kupka has always been a step ahead of me. That was true in 1974 when she first decided to become my patient, and has remained so ever since. She knew about Ignacio Madrazo and his startling claims about brain implants in the treatment of Parkinson's disease long before I did, but that didn't come until almost thirteen years after our first interchange and we'd been through quite a lot by then.

She was thirty-eight years old when I first examined her and she had been a stockbroker or investment counselor for ten years. With her full head of blond hair, bright green eyes, and quick smile, she could easily have passed for thirty or thirty-two. She'd come to see me because she thought she had a neurologic problem and that that problem was most likely Parkinson's disease. For about a year she'd been aware of a tremor of her right hand. It was only evident when her hand was not doing anything—more an embarrassment than a disease. The shaking was most prominent when she was in public, especially when she was with a client. Perhaps it was just her nerves. She had noticed only one other symptom: Her handwriting had deteriorated and become small, tight, tremulous. Writing now took considerable effort and the writing itself was smaller, more cramped.

"That's called micrographia, isn't it?" she asked me.

I nodded. "How do you know that?"

"I've read a great deal about Parkinson's disease. All I can get my hands on. That's how I picked you."

I asked her if she had any other symptoms.

She was not aware of any. There was one other thing that was on her mind.

"What's that?"

"My uncle had Parkinson's. He had a tremor, just like mine. I remember. I was just a kid then. He had surgery, in New York. And he had a stroke during surgery. He was never the same. He got worse and worse. He died before I graduated from high school. I graduated the same year you did."

Clearly a woman who had done her homework.

"But," she went on, "there was so much less doctors could do then. There was no levodopa. Or Sinemet. Or Parlodel."

That was all true, those medicines had revolutionized the treatment of Parkinson's disease. But how did she already know about Parlodel? It was the newest experimental drug then. I'd just started using it in selected patients. I asked her.

"I have my sources."

I then walked Alexa Kupka into one of our examining rooms and examined her. She had been an astute diagnostician. She had three of the four cardinal manifestations of Parkinson's disease and it only takes two to make a firm diagnosis. The four are:

Rest Tremor. A rhythmic abnormal movement of hands and fingers that was more marked at rest than during activity. I didn't have to take her into the exam room to see her tremor. It was there whenever her right hand was at rest.

Rigidity. Stiffness of the limbs, which resist movement and have increased inertia. This requires examination, an actual putting on of the hands. I moved her arms slowly. The resistance was there, the rigidity, and it had the right quality, as if pulling the arm over a racket or cogwheel. The cogwheel rigidity of Parkinson's disease.

Bradykinesia. Literally, this means slow movements. The term encompasses a host of symptoms, from a poverty of spontaneous movements, to difficulty in initiating all voluntary movements, to profound slowness of movements once initiated. One of the hallmarks is the classic slow, small, labored handwriting known as micrographia. She'd already told me about that, but I had her write a few sentences to see it for myself. She did and I saw it. She also had other

166

signs; her right arm didn't swing as she walked and her right leg dragged ever so little. There was a decrease in facial movements. All of her fine finger movements were slowed—not much, but enough to be abnormal. (All that was missing was the *Loss of Postural Reflexes*, imbalance, but that only comes later in the disorder.)

I knew everything I had to know. I completed the rest of a neurologic exam just to prove that there was no evidence of any other neurologic disease. I was confident that there wouldn't be and there wasn't. We walked back to my office and I told her that she had Parkinson's disease and then tried to answer her questions.

Was it hereditary? No.

The literature she had read had not been so definite.

She already had a fairly good understanding of what was happening in her brain. I let her explain it to me. She did extremely well. A small group of nerve cells, or neurons, called the substantia nigra, or black substance, were dying. In fact, most of them had already died.

"Why?" she asked rhetorically. "You scientists don't know," she also answered as I sat back and listened. These neurons make a chemical called dopamine and deliver this dopamine to another part of the brain known as the striatum. As the cells of the substantia nigra die, the amount of dopamine they can deliver declines and that's what causes parkinsonism. The striatum helps control movement, and to do that normally it needs dopamine. Deprived of dopamine, the patient develops tremor, rigidity, and slowness.

She had watched her uncle die after he'd been bedridden for several years. "There is much more that can be done now, isn't there?"

"Of course. We have many powerful medications."

"So you can help me?" The mask of learning had fallen away, revealing a frightened patient.

"Of course," I reassured her.

Would she end up like her uncle? Probably not. We had new and powerful medicines, I repeated, and were developing more every year.

"Parlodel," she intoned.

"Parlodel," I repeated, still wondering how she already knew about Parlodel.

And so our relationship began. I started her on Sinemet, a chemical from which the brain makes the needed dopamine. It worked. Her handwriting improved. Her tremor became less noticeable. She could once again eat in restaurants without embarrassment. Her life as an investment counselor flourished. She changed jobs and moved up to investment banker, taking most, if not all, of her clients with her to her new firm.

The years went by. Her disease progressed, but only slowly. In time, I increased her daily intake of Sinemet. Later we added new medicines. Parlodel. It was about then that she became a partner in her firm. Then along came Permax. She was the one who told me that Eli Lilly was developing Permax, long before I would have heard about it through the usual medical channels. "How do you know all these things?" I asked.

"It's my business to stay a step ahead." She smiled back.

"That's my business, too," I complained.

"Maybe I'm better in my business," she said.

Each therapeutic maneuver helped her. But as the medicines kept working, her disease kept right on progressing. When she was forty-five, she looked her stated age, and by the time she was forty-eight, she looked closer to fifty-five or sixty. It was of little consolation to either of us to know that without these medications, she would also have been bedridden. Her days fell into a routine, a routine of only intermittent good health, of alternating periods of mobility, as her medicine clicked in, and immobility when it failed to work any longer.

6:00 A.M.	First pills of the day.
7:00 A.M.	Mobile enough to get dressed, eat breakfast, and go to work.
8:30 A.M.	Arrive at work. No disability.
10:00 A.M.	Turn off. Immobile. Unable to work.
11:30 A.M.	Back on. Able to work or go out to lunch.
2:00 P.M.	Off. A two-hour nap on a cot in her office.
4:00 P.M.	On.
6:30 P.M.	Home. Half on, half off.
9:00 P.M.	Off.

Day in and day out. We tried everything. We tried all of the newest experimental medications. There was nothing more I could do.

That was in the spring of 1987. She called me one day to discuss the possibility of retiring. Then she called me the next day, all excited. They were doing brain implants in Mexico.

"Who?"

"A neurosurgeon named Madrazo."

It was not a name I had ever heard before. Not that that meant very much. I knew the names of relatively few neurosurgeons since Parkinson's disease had slipped out of their bailiwick long ago.

"And?" I asked.

"His patients are doing brilliantly."

"What kind of implants?"

"Adrenal."

"The Swedes have done a number of these and their patients didn't improve much at all. Those patients were carefully studied by specialists in Parkinson's disease."

"Madrazo's are better. All of them. He apparently has altered the technique."

If it wasn't the same exact operation, then there might well be a reason for excitement. Neurosurgery is not like giving out pills to patients. Technique can be everything. "How many patients?" I asked.

"Half a dozen," she told me.

I was beginning to be impressed. The theory was simple enough. It is easy to move a patient's own tissue from one place in the body to another. What the Swedes had done was put part of one of each patient's own adrenal glands inside that part of the brain that has lost dopamine. Why the adrenal gland? Because it makes dopamine and other dopamine-related chemicals.

"How do you know all of this?"

"I have my sources," she again informed me. One of them was an article that had appeared in the *Los Angeles Times*.

"Not exactly the *New England Journal of Medicine*," I countered.

That she readily admitted.

"When his article appears in the *New England Journal of Medicine,* call me." And then I added far less skeptically, "By then, we might set up a program of our own. You never know."

Less than three months later, she did call me. "It's in the *New England Journal of Medicine*," she said.

"What is?"

"The article by Madrazo, the Mexican neurosurgeon."

"When?" I asked.

"Thursday."

It was only Tuesday, but she had somehow managed to get a preprint prior to publication. How she had managed that I had no idea and Alexa Kupka was not about to tell me. The overall process I understood. The *New England Journal of Medicine* loves publicity, loves exposure, loves making news. In fact, it seems to have become dedicated not just to publishing medical news but also to creating that news. The authors of articles to be published in the *NEJM* are forbidden to discuss their articles, no matter what the subject is, until the *NEJM* itself sends out its preprints to newspapers, TV, and magazines throughout the world. And to Alexa Kupka. And this law applies to all articles, from new treatments for AIDS to Madrazo's implant surgery. It is the *NEJM* that sets up the news releases and makes the headlines.

"Get me a copy," I requested.

She had a messenger deliver one that morning.

In the report, Madrazo described his treatment of two young patients with supposedly "intractable and incapacitating" Parkinson's disease. In both, fragments of each patient's own adrenal gland had been transplanted into their brains. The reported results were spectacular. It was hard not to get excited. More than hard; it was almost impossible. In the first patient, all of the major manifestations of Parkinson's disease had virtually disappeared within ten months. The patient had been transformed from a totally immobilized, all-but-helpless shadow of a man to someone who could play soccer with his twelve-year-old son. In the second patient, the same sort of improvement was seen within three months following the operation. A miracle. A virtual cure.

But my enthusiasm was not unbridled. In part, I admit, it was because of the source. Call it prejudice, but the fact remained that I had heard of neither Madrazo nor his co-authors, and after all, the last major medical advance to come out of Mexico had occurred in 1954 when it was announced that laetrile was *the* cure for cancer. It wasn't just prejudice or skepticism. Madrazo's article had demonstrated a lack of sophisticated knowledge of Parkinson's disease and its proper evaluation and treatment. Madrazo didn't use any of the accepted methods of Parkinson's disease research. He invented his own scale, his own way of evaluating how severe the Parkinson's disease was. Why? There were published scales. Almost all investigators studying Parkinson's disease use these scales to communicate results, so that the readers actually know what is being described. The neurology journals demand this. Did Madrazo even know them? His article showed no evidence of that. Did the editors of *NEJM*? And all the hoopla was based on just two patients, one of whom had only been followed for three months. There were just too many unanswered questions.

Was I just carping? What difference did it make what kind of a scale he used? His patients got better. In ways that no scales were designed to measure. Or needed.

I wasn't the only one who had these misgivings. Many of us who specialize in Parkinson's disease had the same feelings, the same doubts, the same questions. But in the long run, what difference did his method of evaluation make? Were we just jealous, just protecting our turf, our reputations, our careers? What he had done was describe a new technique, a technique that held out hope and promise. Nitpicking was not the right response.

There were questions that had to be answered.

Did the two patients really have "intractable" Parkinson's disease? And "intractable" by whose standards?

Would all Parkinson's disease patients improve? A cure should cure everyone. There should be no preferential miracles. But if not, which patients would respond? And why? And more importantly, which ones would not be cured and why not?

What were the risks?

And how long would the improvement last?

What made our collective doubts worse was that we had all heard rumors. We'd been hearing them for months. Rumors of operations in Mexico City and of wonderful responses. *And* these rumors involved a lot more than just two patients. Alexa Kupka had heard about six patients. So had the *Los Angeles Times*. Others had heard of more. Seven. Eight. How many? Who knew? What had happened to the others?

Had the editors of *NEJM* heard the same rumors? Apparently not.

The editors of the *NEJM* had been so impressed by Madrazo's successes that the same issue which carried his article also contained an editorial calling for the National Institutes of Health to support a clinical trial of this procedure in multiple centers throughout the United States. And the editors of the *NEJM* were not the only ones who were impressed. Parkinson patients throughout the world were electrified. As were their families, and their doctors. A cure for Parkinson's disease had been discovered. *The New York Times* called Madrazo's accomplishment a miracle. Within weeks, they had interviewed Madrazo and several of his patients in Mexico City who had jumped on Madrazo's bandwagon. And why not? Madrazo had the results that were necessary to support his claims. Most of his eighteen patients were almost cured!

Most of the eighteen! This number made believers of the world of patients and media.

He hadn't just operated on two patients. There were far more than two successes. It could not be written off as a couple of flukes. Something was happening. Something important. The enthusiasm was contagious. It was unlike anything I'd seen or felt since the early days of levodopa, the first real breakthrough in the treatment of Parkinson's disease, almost twenty years ago.

The patients all wanted it.

And we wanted to give it to them. And answer the scientific questions while we were at it. How often did it work? If it failed, how often? And why? Yet at the same time we all had our nagging doubts. The added numbers also added to these.

Where had the other patients suddenly come from?

When had they been operated upon?

What had happened to those who had not been cured? This was the only question the *Times* had asked. Three had died. When? Two had died before the *NEJM* article had been published. What ever happened to scientific truth?

I was puzzled. I myself had published several articles in the prestigious *NEJM* over the last two decades. I was well aware of the *NEJM* rule that it will not publish an article if it has been reported anywhere before. Not just in scientific circles, but anywhere: *The New York Times,* the *Los Angeles Times.* It was a rule that had been invoked more than once. In 1976, the *NEJM* rejected the first scientific report of Lyme disease because *The New York Times* had already carried a brief news report of the original verbal presentation, written by a science writer. In 1982, the *NEJM* rejected the first report of AIDS transmitted by a blood transfusion because it had first been published in the Centers for Disease Control's *Morbidity and Mortality Weekly Report*, a report few people ever see.

So, the *NEJM* paid attention to the lay press. It rejected articles because of what appeared in newspapers. It had to know what had appeared in the press. And what appeared was that Madrazo had cribbed the figures. The fact became crystal clear within two months of the *NEJM* article when *The New York Times* reported that he had not operated on two patients, but many more, and that some of them had died. Maybe it didn't change the meaning of his report, the real medical significance. Perhaps his new technique was the miracle we all wanted. But he hadn't played the game honestly. And the *NEJM* has a responsibility to its readers who might not read *The New York Times*, and should have retracted or at least revised its editorial. The

NEJM had fanned the public furor for brain implants. It had a responsibility to bank those flames of enthusiasm. Otherwise every neurosurgeon might start doing implants. For what good? At what risk?

I reread the editorial. The author was not even a Parkinson's disease specialist. He was a neurologist who specialized in pediatric neurology.

I waited for the *NEJM* to say something about Madrazo, to have him explain the real facts, but they published nothing.

Parkinson's disease patients across the world had no such concerns. The patients were interested in medical progress, not editorial carping. They each knew that Madrazo's miraculous procedure would become their own personal miracle. They clamored for the operation. Their clamor fueled a process which came to have a momentum of its own, one which swept us all up.

It became a bandwagon. A bandwagon led by the *NEJM*, but a bandwagon we all jumped upon quite willingly and eagerly. We helped create the momentum.

I never bothered to write a letter to the editor of the *NEJM*. I had more pressing matters to pursue. We had to get our implant program off the ground.

In the United States, there was a mad scramble to be the first to do implants. The race was won by a team of neurosurgeons at Vanderbilt, led by Dr. George Allen. Allen carried out the procedure in a young woman and did it replete with nationally televised press conferences, which long preceded any scientific reports.

We at Rush jumped into the implant business in a big way. We had Madrazo visit us. Our neurosurgeon, Richard Penn, visited him and watched him do a procedure. We designed our protocol and submitted it to our hospital's Committee on Human Investigation for approval, a process that usually takes two to four months. Ten days later, Alexa called. Our project would be approved in two days.

How did she know?

She had her sources. There were, I remembered, nonscientific members on the committee, including clergy, lawyers, and so forth.

She wanted to be one of our patients. Not the first. She'd let us get our feet wet first, and not the last; we might lose interest by then.

"Which one?"

"Four. I want to be the fourth."

"We'll have to see if you meet all of our criteria for patient selection."

"I do," she assured me confidently.

Two days later the approval came through, just as Alexa had promised. We were all set. In June 1987, we did our first implant, our first brain implant.

Brain implant. The phrase itself conjures up images of science fiction. The procedure was anything but that. It's all very straight-forward and combines two fairly standard operations. A general surgeon removed one of the patient's two adrenal glands. Nothing fancy in that. General surgeons do it all the time for patients with various forms of cancers, patients who were a lot sicker than our patients. We asked Dr. Tom Witt, one of our best cancer surgeons, to do that part of the project. He agreed. The adrenal sits atop the kidney and can be reached and removed without damaging the kidney or any other major organ. Once it's removed, the surgeon dissects the gland. The adrenal has two parts: the outer cortex that makes steroids and is of no interest at all in this procedure, and the inner adrenal medulla, which makes adrenalin and dopamine. Dr. Witt separated the two and cut the medulla into small slices. In the meantime our neurosurgeon, Dr. Richard Penn, got the brain ready to receive the medulla. First, he removed some of the bone over the right frontal lobe of the brain. He then passed an ultrasound probe through the substance of the brain. This probe sends out and receives sound much like a miniature radar apparatus. This allows the surgeon to locate different structures deep inside the brain. This, Richard felt, was an improvement on Madrazo's technique. Madrazo didn't use a probe, he did his freehand. Our technique was safer and more reliable. The target was the major fluid-filled cavity (the ventricle) deep inside the brain and the striatum just below it. Once he had found the striatum, Dr. Penn removed a small part of it and then packed the small pieces of the adrenal medulla into the resulting cavity.

That's it. The implant procedure is all over. Except for the waiting. Madrazo's patients did not improve immediately. Neither did ours.

The events of the next year are all etched into my mind as individual occurrences, yet the whole remains somewhat of a blur. It's a time that is hard to recreate, a time of excitement, of discovery, of doubt, of hope, of fear, of pressure. So much pressure. I, fortunately, kept my weekly notes to preserve my perspective on looking back.

June. We performed our first two implant procedures. No miracles. At four weeks post-op, we could not see any improvement. Then the patients began to notice something. Their amount of down time was less. Less "off" time. More "on" time.

174

July. Patients one and two reported continued improvement. Operation number three took place. Then operation number four. Alexa Kupka. She still wanted us to do it. She all but demanded it.

We still had our doubts. I told her about them and about all the rumors. Many of us were increasingly skeptical of the glowing reports coming out of Mexico. Some of the patients Madrazo had considered successes were far from that. One was being followed in California by a friend of mine. Another in Miami. Both had been surgical disasters.

"If it was good enough for the *New England Journal of Medicine*, its good enough for me." And in a way, for us, too.

So, Dr. Richard Penn and Dr. Tom Witt did their bit and it all went well.

By then, more and more procedures were being done, both in Mexico and across the United States. More than fifteen centers had started programs. Some were logical places with expertise in caring for and evaluating Parkinson's disease. Others were not. Just neighborhood neurosurgeons performing local miracles.

August. We organized a national meeting in Chicago of all investigators interested in performing implants on Parkinson's disease patients. We presented the results on our first four patients. They were all somewhat better. Not cured, not miracles, but the patients were better. They had more "on" time and less "off" time. Less bad time and the bad time was not as bad. Alexa was no longer talking of retiring. Instead of a pair of two-hour periods each day during which she was immobile, her "off" phases lasted only an hour apiece and during them she could still walk by herself. She no longer had to end her day at nine but could stay up until eleven. She hadn't done that in years. Her "on" time was not much better, but even before surgery that had been pretty good.

Others presented their results. Some were similar to ours. Others were a litany of surgical disaster, of postoperative complications, of deaths, of permanent neurologic catastrophes. Often from places with no real experience in treating patients with Parkinson's disease, places that only became interested because of the bandwagon started by Madrazo.

At that meeting it was agreed that small individual studies would not give us the answers we needed. What was needed was cooperative studies with rigid selection criteria, rigid evaluation of patients by neurologists who knew how to evaluate patients using standardized techniques. There was also a need for a registry of as many operated patients as possible. Only these approaches would answer the real questions. How well did the patients do? For how long? And how safe was it? We still had no answers to those questions.

September and October. Alexa Kupka was working full-time. She had the cot removed from her office.

We did another procedure. Number five.

The scientific community was beginning to raise some doubts. Many scientists felt that we were acting prematurely. That we had jumped the gun. More work should have been done on animals. Perhaps we had moved too quickly, but what choice had we had? Madrazo had thrown down a challenge that had to be pursued. Besides, our patients were improving. Success was ours and success was intoxicating. I went to Sweden and presented our results to the pioneers in brain implants.

Coals to Newcastle?

They were impressed.

The day I got back, a physician from Pennsylvania was flown in to see us. He had Parkinson's disease. He'd been treating himself for years. He'd seen an article in the *New England Journal of Medicine*, left his office after a full day of work, went off to Mexico City to see Madrazo, and within days had undergone the surgery and had been confused ever since. He'd had a severe brain injury. A major surgical complication. Could we help him? After all, his surgery had been such a success. Who said that? Madrazo. Was he certain of that? Yes. Yet this physician could no longer practice medicine. He had been in a nursing home ever since he'd flown home.

We did our seventh, and last, implant in February. Why did we stop at seven? We didn't need to do any more. We had set up the needed collaborative studies that along with our results would tell us what we needed to know. And we already knew the most important answer. Parkinson's disease had not been cured. Not in any of our patients or in anyone else's. Except, perhaps, Madrazo's.

March. We hosted the second meeting of all investigators interested in performing implants on Parkinson's disease patients. Again, several teams reported partial benefits following adrenal implants. These paralleled our results. The similarity of the observations was striking. The implants obviously had a beneficial effect. That was evident. But enough to be worth all the risk?

On Sunday morning, Madrazo arrived to give his summary of what he had accomplished. He told us about his thirty-five patients.

Was that all? Was that the entire number? Was he making a full disclosure?

He said he was.

Many were skeptical.

All of his patients were "greatly improved."

All?

All

That question and answer were repeated several times.

And they were "junger," he said. "Much junger."

"Junger," I repeated to myself, "junger." He meant younger.

"You mean they look younger?" I said, hoping to clear the air of our resentment that I could feel building up.

"No. Not look. They are. They are all junger."

My God, I thought, he really believes it. He believes that his patients are younger. A used-car salesman who believes what he says, every single word of it. And we'd all bought a car from him.

From there, the conference deteriorated. Physicians from around the country asked Madrazo about specific patients on whom he'd operated. Patients they had seen. The physician from Pennsylvania.

"His Parkinson's is better," Madrazo told us all. "He is better." That operation had been a success.

Then he was asked about a woman from California who had been in a nursing home in a chronic vegetative state since the surgery. She was all but in a coma.

"Yes, but her Parkinson's is better."

Could he really believe that? He said it. I heard it. So did all the others who were there.

He then went on to describe his experiments in rats. They, too, were younger.

Science covered our meeting. They even quoted me extensively. I had told them that the United States results were "clearly not as spectacular as people thought they would be," and I concluded by pointing out that the disparity between what we were seeing in the American patients and what we had been told about the Mexican patients was "substantial." I didn't mention the patients being "junger."

The *New England Journal of Medicine* remained silent. Silence must be golden.

The story has not ended. Science has moved on. We no longer do those adrenal implants.

Why not?

Not just because there were no miracles, but in part because we now know more. More good, basic research has been completed, research that tried to figure out why such implants have any effect at all. It's not because the adrenal cells survive in the brain and made dopamine. The fact is they don't survive and don't make dopamine. So why did they work? Probably because they produced something, a growth factor perhaps, that made the patient's own injured cells grow. Now we are doing implants with adrenal tissue and a piece of the patient's own nerve that produces nerve-growth factor. Will that be the answer? Perhaps.

And others are implanting fetal nigra cells. Fetal cells, when implanted, do survive and they do produce dopamine.

And many labs are trying to find a specific growth factor for those neurons affected in Parkinson's disease. Does it exist? Will we find it? Will it work? That's what research is all about.

And without Madrazo, we might not have gotten this far. Certainly, not this soon.

We are still following six of our seven patients. One died. Was his death related to our surgery? Probably. One out of seven. Not Alexa. She was better for about three years. Now she's had to retire. She bought three years; for her it was well worth it.

Was it overall?

I'm not convinced. Certainly not for those patients who died in hospitals that weren't really set up to study Parkinson's disease, where nothing was learned except that neurosurgery can be dangerous. And these operations only took place because of Madrazo's article in the *New England Journal of Medicine*.

Alexa and I debate this subject often. Once, I told her what my son had said when I told him about Madrazo.

"Why," he asked, "would anyone go someplace where you can't drink the water to have experimental neurosurgery?" To him that made no sense.

"That's not the question," she said. "Patients are desperate. The question is why you scientists went to a place where you can't drink the water to bring back a miracle? Are you that desperate?"

"The *New England Journal of Medicine* left us with no other choice," I said, knowing that was only part of the answer.

PART FOUR

Adventures in the Medical Trade

I thought of writing books myself once. I had the ideas: I even made notes. But I was a doctor, married with children. You can only do one thing well: Flaubert knew that. Being a doctor was what I did well.*

Julian Barnes
Flaubert's Parrot

18

BELLING THE CAT

Pondering the singular chain of events called "the Krebiozen controversy," I have often recalled a favorite fable of my childhood, a fable about a group of mice who found their community victimized by a stealthy cat. As I recall the story, the mice held a sort of town meeting to discuss the problem. One of their number brightly suggested that all they had to do to prevent the cat from sneaking up on them was to have it wear a bell around its neck. As the mice rejoiced over this simple solution, one of their wise elders rose to ask the devastating question: "But who will bell the cat?"

Patricia Spain Ward, 1984

Once I've introduced myself to a new patient and whoever may be with him, I always ask the same question. I don't ask what the major medical problem is, the chief complaint in medical jargon. That's what we were all taught to do in medical school. Chief Complaint followed by History of Present Illness. CC then HPI. That comes later. "And what is it precisely that brings you to see me?" I ask.

I get a host of different responses. Many have been referred by their physician for a diagnosis or for management of their specific neurologic disorder. Others come on their own for the same reasons, or just to get a second or third opinion on their diagnosis. Knowing the purpose helps me to understand what the patient chooses as his CC and also helps me structure the content of the HPI.

Walter Pipp's reply was most unusual. He did not want a second opinion. He had ALS, amyotrophic lateral sclerosis, and he knew it. He had seen more than a dozen neurologists in half a dozen cities—New York, Boston, Cleveland, Washington, Philadelphia, and Chicago. He had ALS. He even understood what ALS was: a progressive disease of the motor system in which specific nerve cells in the brain and spinal cord, the cells that control movement, start dying off and cause progressive weakness and eventually death. All that he understood.

I nodded.

He also knew that there was no accepted form of treatment.

So why had he come to see me? He knew the diagnosis. He realized the prognosis. He accepted the fact that there was nothing I could do to treat him. Why?

"I want you to be my doctor here at home in case there are any complications."

"Complications from what?"

"Snake venom."

To me, the use of snake venom to treat ALS was a sophisticated form of charlatanism. A twentieth-century version of snake oil, with just enough of a pseudoscientific rationale to give it a thin veneer of respectability. Some neuroscientists have hypothesized the nerve cells die in ALS because they become exhausted from too much uncontrolled stimulation. An interesting theory. Death from excessive excitatory stimulation. But caused by what? Such a state of continuous excessive excitation could be caused by the uncontrolled release of high levels of excitatory neurotransmitters, those chemicals that normally carry messages to other nerve cells. Too much excitation. Too often. And for far too long. Excitatory cell death. If that were true, then a drug which blocked the excitation might slow the rate of cell death. And some snake venoms, in part, kill by causing paralysis as a result of their ability to block the activity of some, but not all, excitatory neurotransmitters in some, but not all, motor nerve cells.

Ergo: A Cure.

Walter Pipp was no fool. He was well educated, a senior vice-president in one of the largest banks in Chicago. He had something to do with commercial real estate, hence his frequent business trips throughout the United States. It was on these that he had visited a wide range of neurologists and learned more about ALS and his future than he wanted to know. He even knew enough not to refer to it by its popular eponym, Lou Gehrig's disease, rejected as parochial by the international scientific community.

I then took a history of his illness from him and examined him. The neurologists had all been correct, Walter Pipp had ALS. He'd had it for about a year. He had mild weakness of both legs and his left arm. He could still lead a fairly normal life, but his voice was just becoming a bit slurred. That was a bad sign. How long did he have to live? It was hard to tell. A year. Two. Perhaps three.

I, of course, had nothing that I could do that could change that.

He did. There was a doctor in Louisiana, not a neurologist, a GP. He was using snake venom to treat ALS.

From what snake?

Pipp didn't know.

Was it purified?

He had no idea.

What was the doctor's name?

Pipp wouldn't tell me.

I didn't push him.

What did he want from me?

The doctor in Louisiana was not a neurologist. I was. That doctor was not here in Chicago. I was. He needed a neurologist here to monitor him, to take care of him if anything went awry. And . . . . He hesitated.

"And what?" I insisted.

"To prove that the snake venom works."

I now understood why he'd come to me.

"You will test me. You will observe me. It works, I know that it does. I've talked to other patients, but none of you scientists believe in it. Why not?"

It was, I realized, a rhetorical question. He didn't want my answer. He didn't want to hear that anecdotal individual testimony does not constitute scientific fact.

"I'll tell you why. Because one of your respected in-group scientists didn't do it, but some hick-town GP who doesn't really know ALS from MS But it works. In both ALS and MS, too."

I shuddered.

"Are you like all the rest? A closed mind, or are you willing to judge for yourself?"

I was willing, on one condition. If it didn't work, he would go public and denounce it through such avenues as patient newsletters and other underground sources of patient information. If it worked, I'd publish it in my journal.

The deal was struck.

As he left, he thanked me and then said, "If you'd been here in 1951, cancer would have been cured."

"Cancer?" I said.

"Krebiozen," he answered.

It was a word I hadn't heard or thought about in twenty years. Krebiozen had been the greatest cancer hoax in the history of the United States. Bigger in its day and better promoted or orchestrated than laetrile. It had started in Chicago and had, at least in my mind, more than a few similarities to the snake venom business on which he was now embarking.

"Krebiozen worked. I know it did." With that, he left. He was to come back in four weeks, two weeks after completing his first two-week course of snake venom bites or injections or whatever.

Krebiozen had been introduced in Chicago in 1951. I was in grammar school then and far more interested in the Chicago White Sox than in cancer. I had heard about it off and on during my career, but was certain of only one detail. The scam succeeded as well as it had because one real scientist, Dr. Andrew Ivy, a renowned name in Chicago medicine gave it credibility. Was I to become the Andrew Ivy of snake venom? And what did I know about Ivy? He'd given my medical school class a series of boring lectures in 1959. But little else.

I needed more details so I retreated to the library. Not to do research on ALS or snake venom—those were subjects I was up on—but to read about Krebiozen.

Krebiozen had been discovered by a Yugoslavian-born physician named Stevan Durovic. He and his brother Marco Durovic had manufactured munitions during World War II—in Yugoslavia—and had somehow managed to escape with money, traveling eventually to Argentina with papal passports.

Those facts aroused all my prejudices. To get out of Yugoslavia with money enough to buy a Vatican passport in 1945 meant one thing to me. The Durovics must have collaborated with the Nazis. Who else ended up in Argentina on papal visas? Papal passports didn't come cheap. And Argentina was not exactly a haven for Yugoslav patriots.

Once in Argentina, Marco established an institute named the Duga Biological Institute, where Stevan Durovic apparently carried out experiments to find a cure for cancer. It was here that he discovered Krebiozen. He never told how, since he was afraid his work would fall into the hands of the Communists who, he claimed, had destroyed the rest of his family.

The Durovics came to Chicago in 1949. Stevan at first attempted to interest faculty members at Northwestern University in a substance of his called Cositerin, which he said treated or cured high blood pressure. When tests there failed to confirm his findings, he came to Ivy at Illinois with a substance (some say the same substance), which he claimed cured cancer. Ivy shared Durovic's theories about the possibility of stimulating natural resistance to tumor growth as a way of treating and perhaps curing cancer, and his hatred of communism.

Ivy had been fifty-eight then. He was in his late sixties when he lectured to my class. He was a scientist with a worldwide reputation. He'd been the Nathan Smith Davis Professor of Physiology and Pharmacology at Northwestern for twenty years before becoming chief executive officer at the University of Illinois School of Medicine in 1946. He was founder and director of the Naval Medical Research Institute during World War II. He'd been executive director of the National Advisory Cancer Council from 1947 to 1951. He'd also been one of the medical consultants at the Nuremberg Trials of War Crimes and was the author of the Nuremberg Code of ethics for human experimentation, and he'd had more than his share of honors, having been at one time or another elected president of a variety of societies, including the Society of Internal Medicine, the American Gastroenterological Association, and the American Physiological Society, among other organizations. This was the man who, as I recalled it, had been snookered by Durovic.

Eighteen months after first meeting Durovic, Ivy publicly announced that clinical trials had convinced him that Krebiozen caused a reduction in tumor size; that when given to cancer patients, it restored their appetite, their ability to sleep, and their sense of well-being; and that it sometimes enabled the bedridden to move about or even return to work.

To any skeptical or even objective observer, all but the first observation sounded much more like decreased depression than a specific effect on the cancer. And nothing was said about increased survival. That, of course, was the real issue. And this was not said through the medium of a peer-reviewed scientific publication, but at a press conference held in Chicago at the Drake Hotel.

I was dumbfounded. How could any real scientist announce anything like this publicly before it had gone through rigorous testing and appropriate peer review? This was not data. This was not science. There had been no statistical analysis. No scientific review. No double-blind studies, just the impressions of a noted scientist. That and testimonials of a few patients. Not all, just some.

Snake oil.

Snake venom.

It was the journalists who used the word cure.

Ivy knew that more work had to be done. He called for widespread testing in many centers throughout the country. This call came not from some corner medical huckster but from a scientist who had helped formulate the National Cancer Institute's guidelines for testing potential anticancer drugs and who had recently helped expose a well-known cancer quack. Ivy's recommendation brought an immediate response.

To the lay press and most of the public, it mattered little that Ivy made his announcement and distributed his brochure of case histories not to a scientific gathering, but to an invited group of newspapermen, drug-house officials, businessmen, physicians, and politicians. Among those present were Chicago Mayor Martin Kennelly, State Attorney John Boyle, and Park Livingston, president of the University of Illinois Board of Trustees, an elected body susceptible to the powerful political currents for which Illinois is noted. Although invited, Governor Adlai Stevenson and Senator Paul Douglas did not attend. Ivy said that he had chosen this time and manner to announce Krebiozen because Senator Paul Douglas, who had long been a close friend, had told him that he must create a dramatic and public demonstration of Krebiozen's real potential, because with such a demonstration, Douglas could convince Congress to grant citizenship to the Durovics, whose Vatican papers would soon expire.

Back to the Durovics and their papal travel documents.

Was that what was behind it all? The Durovics' need not to lose their visas and have to go back to Yugoslavia? It worked. Douglas was right. Once the announcement was made and the furor began, Stevan and his brother Marco got their citizenship by a special act of Congress, putting them in a class with Winston Churchill and Raoul Wallenberg. Why not Fidel Castro?

A non-profit Krebiozen Research Foundation was founded with Ivy as its president, while the Durovics set up their own pharmaceutical company.

Walter Pipp came back to see me as scheduled, four weeks after our first appointment. He was thrilled by his improvement. He had had two weeks of injections and they were working. He felt stronger, he fatigued less easily, he slept better, he felt better. He was thinking of helping to set up a venture-capital company to manufacture and distribute the snake venom. It could be made by genetically engineered bacteria. Or perhaps a nonprofit research foundation. Or both. Selkirk, Dr. Selkirk, the physician who was treating him, thought that the latter was a better idea. Selkirk Pharmaceuticals and the Lou Gehrig Society, or something similar.

186

Finally he quieted down and I was able to examine him. His neurological exam was no different. True, he was no worse, but that was not unusual; the progression of ALS is often so slow that the physician cannot see any evidence of change in just four weeks. The important observation was that he was no better. The key findings on neurologic examination showed no evidence of improvement. His weakness was unchanged. His loss of muscle mass, what we call atrophy of the muscles, was no different. His muscles still twitched spontaneously. These little twitches, which are not enough to move a joint but look like the twitches of muscle under a horse's skin, are evidence of active disease of the motor neurons and are sometimes said to represent those motor cells waving goodbye. Walter Pipp's were still waving. I was done.

"I'm so much better."

"I'm glad you feel better," I said, being noncommittal but as supportive as I could. He did feel better, like Ivy's patients, and in the same ways. Less fatigued, sleeping better, a greater sense of well-being. Not any increase in a specific muscle activity. Not a better grip. Or an ability to walk faster. All nonspecific vague feelings. He did feel better. He no longer knew he was dying. He was no longer without hope. There was a treatment and he was getting it and he felt better. His depression had lifted. It was gone. He had hope for a future.

"You're going to have to write that article," he reminded me.

"I hope so. It's still a bit early to start it."

"Perhaps for you but not for me."

"What's that mean?"

He smiled back.

"You're not about to give public testimonial to other patients?"

"No. No testimonials to other patients."

I was relieved.

Walter Pipp was scheduled to go back for another course of treatments that week. I'd see him again in another four weeks.

Ivy had remained adamant in his support of Krebiozen. Cancer could be cured. A final solution was just around the corner. Others were not so convinced. The *Journal of the American Medical Association* soon published a "Status Report on Krebiozen." The report started with a standard disclaimer about the need for authentic information, for real data, not just testimonials or anecdotes. What the AMA committee called "tremendous world wide public interest" had, they felt, created a "moral obligation" which in their opinion transcended the usual ethical strictures against the testing of "secret remedies." The body of the report stated that Krebiozen had no effect in a hundred cancer patients at six locations around the country, one-third of them at the University of Illinois' Tumor Clinic. Ivy counter-attacked. The report was not based on controlled clinical trials. It was unscientific. It proved nothing.

Ivy's attack was pathetic. He was right, of course. The studies had not been rigidly controlled. They had not been blind. Just like his own studies. Except more patients had been studied and this report was making no unsubstantiated claims.

The argument dragged on for years. In the end, Durovic fled to Switzerland to avoid prosecution for income tax evasion. It seemed that, at least according to the IRS, much of the money raised by the Krebiozen Research Foundation ended up in Durovic's own pocket. Ivy was later charged with some forty-nine counts of failure to comply with federal drug laws regulating experimental drugs. And of course, no evidence ever demonstrated that Krebiozen (which turned out to be nothing more than creatinine, a normal constituent of everyone's urine, a breakdown product of protein metabolites) ever cured anyone of anything, much less that it changed the natural history of cancer. As one of my teachers put it, when Durovic started out, the life expectancy of acute leukemia in an adult was ninety days. Days! He gave such patients Krebiozen. Well, he didn't really give it. The patients purchased it from the Krebiozen Research Foundation. And because of the Krebiozen, the patient lived for months. Three to be exact. Three months.

Not days, but months.

Such was the monumental therapeutic effect of Krebiozen on acute leukemia.

Four weeks later, Walter Pipp once again came bounding into my office. He could not contain his excitement.

We talked. Or rather, he talked. He'd finished his second course of snake venom injections and he was so much better. He had so much more energy. He knew he was cured. Or if not cured, he'd turned the tide. The course of his disease had been reversed.

A cure of ALS.

If Lou Gehrig were still alive, he could still be playing first base for the New York Yankees.

"What's better?" I asked.

"Everything," he informed me, conveying no real information.

I knew he felt better. He was less depressed. He had hope, faith, confidence.

But was anything really better? Had any of his specific symptoms decreased? The dragging of his feet? The weakness of his hand? "What specifically?" I persisted.

"Everything. Can't you tell?" he countered. "Examine me. See for yourself. Here, watch me walk." With that he jumped out of the chair and bounded down the hall to the examining room. He bounded with the enthusiasm of a kid who had just hit his first home run and the foot drop of a patient with ALS, for his left foot was weaker. When he lifted the left leg, the left foot did not elevate normally. It dropped down and dragged along the floor, scraping the rug, scuffing his shoe.

He had not had a foot drop four weeks earlier. He was progressing.

The rest of the exam revealed little more. Nothing was improved. Not the weakness. Not the atrophy. Not the fasciculations. They, in fact, were spreading. For the first time, I observed some in his face. His disease had turned no corner. No tide had been turned.

"See," he said, "now you know."

What could I say? I knew what I knew, but what purpose could possibly be served by stripping him of all hope.

"You ready to write that article?" he continued.

"I'm sharpening my pencil," I replied. "But it's still early."

"I know. I have two more courses to go."

"No testimonials yet, either."

"No," he smiled.

I decided to take a different tact. "Why are you so certain that Krebiozen worked?"

"It cured my dad."

"Your dad?"

"Yes. He was a patient here. In this very hospital. He had a lymphoma. Hodgkin's disease. It was incurable then. He got Krebiozen. He was one of the first. Cured. One hundred percent. It even cured his epilepsy. He died last year of a stroke. They did an autopsy. He had no evidence of Hodgkin's. None at all. No one ever published that. A proven cure from Krebiozen."

"What was his name?" I asked.

"Pipp. Wallace Pipp."

"Where was the autopsy done?"

"Here."

I nodded. A cure from Krebiozen. A cure of Hodgkin's disease.

It was worth looking into.

It was easier to get information on Wallace Pipp than I had thought it would be. I called pathology and got Mark Koenig. He as the director of gross pathology and in charge of all autopsies. He had performed the autopsy on Wallace Pipp. Pipp had died of a cerebral hemorrhage, a massive stroke with bleeding directly into the brain itself. The bleeding, as always, had been the result of many years of high blood pressure. All in all, a far too common occurrence and nothing out of the ordinary. Why had I called?

"He'd had Hodgkin's."

"He had no evidence of Hodgkin's on post," Koenig informed me.

That's what his son had already told me. "A cure?" I suggested.

"Yes." He agreed.

"From Krebiozen." I added.

"From what?" Koenig was too young to know what I was talking about, so I told him the entire story

Koenig was interested, but skeptical. "Where was he diagnosed?" he asked me.

"Here, I think."

"We never throw anything away. I'll check."

Two weeks later Koenig called me back. He had found the original biopsy material. Pipp had been diagnosed as having Hodgkin's in 1950.

"Right before the Krebiozen business," I said. "There was no effective treatment then, unless it was localized to the neck."

"He had generalized disease with enlarged lymph nodes everywhere."

"And you found none at post?"

"None."

"So he was cured by Krebiozen?"

"Not quite. And he's already been published by your own department."

I understood. He hadn't been cured by Krebiozen. He'd never even had Hodgkin's. Not real Hodgkin's disease. Enlargement of the lymph nodes that resembles Hodgkin's disease is a rare side effect of drugs used to treat epilepsy. Wallace Pipp had had epilepsy. He developed enlarged lymph nodes. One was biopsied. A diagnosis of Hodgkin's was made. Today we'd stop his medication, but back in 1950 this rare side effect was not well known. So he was told he had

190

a fatal disease. A disease we could not cure. One we could not even treat. He became desperate. He stopped taking his medications. He went to see Ivy as soon as he heard about Krebiozen.

One shot and he was cured.

No more lymph node enlargement. No more Hodgkin's.

Two years later, he went to see one of our neurologists. Should he go back on his anticonvulsants?

Had he had any seizures?

No.

Then there was no reason to take anticonvulsants.

His case history, without any mention of Krebiozen, was later published as part of a short series of three patients who had had a Hodgkin's-like state from anticonvulsants, in whom discontinuation of the medications had "cured" the disorder.

Had the others also thought they'd been cured by Krebiozen? Had they gotten Krebiozen? No. The other two had been "cured" before Durovic came to Chicago.

So much for Wallace Pipp's cure. How about Walter?

He bounded into my office for his next visit a bit less unabashedly. His enthusiasm was not quite as manic. "I've almost got this thing licked," he told me.

His foot drop was more marked. I found more weakness wherever I looked for it and more atrophy. And more fasciculations. More nerve cells saying their last goodbyes.

All he had now was his enthusiasm and his hope. Those I had to leave intact. I could not rob him of those. I asked no probing questions. I sought out no specific details.

I just asked one question. "Have you given any testimonials for Dr. Selkirk?"

"No," he said with a sigh. "But keep your pencils sharpened."

I said that I would.

As he left, he gave me a business card. I didn't read it until after he'd left. It was a card for Selkirk Pharmaceuticals. Walter Pipp was listed as Chairman of the Board of Directors.

About a month later, I saw Walter Pipp for the last time. This time he shuffled into my office. He no longer had one foot drop; now both feet dragged against the rug. His voice, too, had changed. It was no longer loud and crisp, but softer and with a slur that was apparent to the trained ear of a neurologist.

I asked him how he was.

"Wonderful!"

I was in awe.

"Cured. And spreading the word."

Spreading the word! To other patients?

No.

Thank God.

"Not yet," he said softly.

"Not yet?"

"I have other work to do."

"What other work?"

"I'm raising venture capital for Selkirk Pharmaceuticals. We need twenty-five million. We already have eight. That means I've only got to raise another seventeen. Really only sixteen. I'm going to put in another one."

"Another one million?"

"I wish I had more. It's the opportunity of a lifetime."

"For whom?"

"Me. You. Everyone. A cure for ALS. And Alzheimer's. Selkirk told me all about that. It's a secret, but I can tell you. You and the investors."

Shades of the Durovic brothers.

"How can you do that?"

"How can I not? It's my duty. I'm cured."

"You're not cured."

"You are like all of the others," he started. "All those who condemned Krebiozen," he slurred at me. "It saved my father."

"No it didn't."

"I don't believe you."

I told him the entire story. I even showed him a copy of the article. He remained unconvinced. I had to convince him.

"My father lived for thirty-eight years because of Krebiozen. And I'll live that long, too. Not because of you, but because of Selkirk and his serum. It's the elixir of life, the life of brain cells."

I had to stop him.

"I'm cured. So will all the others be with ALS, Alzheimer's, MS."

"You're dying. You know it. I know it. Selkirk knows it. That snake venom doesn't cure a goddamned thing. Not ALS. Not Alzheimer's. Not MS. It's as worthless as Krebiozen."

He got up and started to shuffle slowly out of my office, dragging one foot after the other.

"Junk," I said. "Don't throw away your money."

He said nothing.

"Don't swindle others."

"Krebiozen cured my father. Durovic was a great scientist."

"A great swindler," I said, "who fled to Switzerland rather than face charges here."

He said nothing more.

I never saw Walter Pipp again. He was dead in less than four months. I learned about it when I read his obituary in the *Chicago Tribune*. The obituary made no mention of Selkirk Pharmaceuticals. I later learned that Pipp had dissolved the venture and returned all the money two days before he died. I learned that from another patient of mind who had invested money when Pipp had told him that I agreed that the venom had cured him.

"Why didn't you call me?"

"I couldn't."

"Why not?"

"You never tell one patient about another patient."

"True."

"And he was cured. He told me so himself."

I'd made the only choice I could. I'd robbed Pipp of all hope. I'd left him with nothing. All he had was the truth and the inexorable progression of his ALS. He, too, had made the right choice.

Would he have lived longer had I not robbed him of that hope? There is no proof one way or the other. Do prayers work? Is there any proof? Can there ever be? Science will never know.

But in my heart, I think I shortened his life. I'm sure of that. As certain as I am that the snake venom was useless, that Selkirk was a charlatan. That Durovic was a charlatan. That Krebiozen never cured anyone. And that robbed of hope, Walter Pipp gave up and died.

Thanks to me.

19

Other People's Patients

"Most Welshmen are worthless,
an inferior breed, doctor."
He did not know I was Welsh.
Then he praised the architects
of the German death-camps—
did not know I was a Jew.
He called liberals, "White blacks,"
and continued to invent curses.

When I palpated his liver
I felt the soft liver of Goering;
When I lifted my stethoscope
I heard the heartbeats of Himmler;
when I read his encephalograph
I thought, "Sieg Heil, Mein Fuhrer."

In the clinic's dispensary
red berry of black bryony,
cowbane, deadly nightshade, deathcap.
Yet I prescribed for him
as if he were my brother.

Later that night I must have slept
on my arm: momentarily
my right hand lost its cunning.

Dannie Abse
"Case History"

PASTEUR'S PATIENT

Rabies. Even today the name strikes fear in the minds of patients and physicians alike. The imagined scenario is always the same: A person is bitten by a rabid dog, sometimes a rabid wild animal, then the disease strikes, weeks to months later. And the disease itself is frightening both to the patient and anyone who sees him. The patient is reduced to an uncontrolled nervous system, to a series of grotesque, uncontrolled contortions, a succession of painful spasms racking the body and the soul, resulting finally in the salvation of insanity, coma, and death. For in the end, the patient always dies. Rabies is 100 percent fatal. It cannot be treated as such. No antibiotics help, no antiviral agents. But for over a hundred years, it has been preventable, thanks to the work of the world's first microbiologist, Louis Pasteur. Pasteur, one of the great names in the history of medicine, was not a physician; he was trained to be a chemist. His original work had nothing to do with the diseases of mankind. His career was in horticulture. His field was the study of the diseases that plagued French winegrowers. But diseases are diseases, whether they are the diseases of plants or man, and the commonest diseases that attack large numbers of individuals, men or plants, are infectious, so Pasteur became not just a chemist but also a bacteriologist and over time his horizon expanded from diseases of plants to those of animals. His list of accomplishments is staggering. In retrospect, his evolution from pure chemistry to bacteriology and then immunology seems quite logical. To contemporary nineteenth-century eyes, it was revolutionary.

All in all, Pasteur made at least six outstanding contributions to the fields of chemistry, bacteriology, and industrial chemistry. His first major accomplishment was in his original discipline, chemistry, and was completed in 1848, when Pasteur was only twenty-six years of age. Pasteur was studying tartaric acid crystals under the microscope. He studied the relationship of those carbon-containing (organic) crystals to polarized light, demonstrating the existence of two forms of rotatory activity, to the left or to the right. Levorotatory or dextrorotary. A basic division of all organic substances. A basic division that is still one of the major cardinal principles of the entire field of organic chemistry.

His study of fermentation of alcohol and of lactic acid in sour milk six years later led him to the concept that such fermentation was caused by living organisms and that these organisms were introduced by air and were not spontaneously generated. The issue of spontaneous generation had been a controversial subject in science for over a century. Pasteur came out solidly against spontaneous generation and performed experiments that help answer the question once and for all. He demonstrated this by boiling an infusion in an open flask with the observation that putrefaction then occurred. However, if the boiling was done after the flask had been hermetically sealed, the solution remained pure. No putrefaction occured. This was the crucial experiment that suggested the possibility of anti-sepsis to Lister some eleven years later.

Pasteur later saved the French wine industry by finding that souring of wine was due to parasitic growths and that these could be destroyed by heating the wine for a few minutes at a temperature of 50 to 60° Celsius. This process was developed in 1864 and has been extended to other fields, including the purification of milk, and is still known today as pasteurization. He was able to rescue the French silk industry in 1865. Silkworms were shriveling up and dying by the hundreds of thousands. If this continued there would soon be no French silk industry. But what was killing them off? No one knew. Pasteur soon learned that the silkworms in France all were being fed damp mulberry leaves and that these damp mulberry leaves were often covered with spots. It wasn't the silkworms that were diseased; it was the mulberry leaves. And of course, not by spontaneous generation. Prevention of spread of the *vibrion* to mulberry leaves would save the silkworm. And it did. He eliminated the disease, ended the plague.

His major contributions involved diseases of animals, diseases that only occasionally involved humans. The first was anthrax. Anthrax can at times infect people but it is primarily a disease of sheep and cattle and as such can have a major economic impact. In the 1870s, anthrax was decimating the French sheep and wool industry. Solving this problem next attracted Pasteur's attention and once that was solved he was attracted to another disease of animals, man's old scourge, rabies. And rabies, of course, is not primarily a disease of man, man only gets it accidentally when bitten by a rabid animal, usually a dog. It was a disease of dogs—or at least that was what Pasteur believed.

Pasteur worked at the time when bacteriology was just coming of age, and the first principle of bacteriology was to find the responsible bacteria. That was easier said than done, but the steps of the process were known. These steps are now called Koch's postulates, after the German bacteriologist Robert Koch, who first demonstrated the usefulness of this approach. The postulates are straightforward enough and still apply:

1) The microorganism must be demonstrated in every case of the disease.
2) The microorganism must be cultivated in pure culture.
3) The microorganism must then be inoculated from that cul-

ture to a susceptible animal and must produce the same disease.

4) The microorganism must be recovered from the animals that have been infected by it.

Using this process, Koch discovered the tuberculous bacillus, the cause of tuberculosis, the white plague of mankind, as well as the cholera vibrio, the cause of epidemics of cholera, and the bacillus of bubonic plague. The first step was always the same, discovery of the bacteria. Isolate it, identify it, see it under the microscope. But rabies is not caused by a bacterium. It is caused by a virus, a virus that could not be seen and could not be isolated, an agent whose presence could only be proved by the result of that presence, the occurrence of disease. This had not been the case with anthrax. Pasteur had seen the anthrax bacillus long before he had isolated it and then developed a vaccine for it. The rabies virus he never saw. But as a chemist, he did not let this divert him from his goal. He didn't know that he had to isolate the cause to prevent the effect. He just went on ahead and did it.

Pasteur set about to solve the problem with his usual energy, imagination, and tenacity. Even though the virus could not be seen, Pasteur bypassed these steps and went on next to postulate injecting various infected tissue into healthy animals, and observing these animals for the development of the disease. A blind passage from animal to animal, from rabid dog to normal, healthy dogs. And the dogs developed rabies. With this method, Pasteur proved that the unseen culprit had to be present in saliva, nerves, spinal cord, and brain. His next job was to produce a vaccine. He now knew the entire life cycle of the virus. Once spread through the saliva of an infected animal, the virus travels through the nerves to the spinal cord and then to the brain. The slowness of its journey through the nerves accounts for the variable period at which the disease develops after the bite. It takes weeks or even months to arrive at the brain, and in its course it does not disturb the function of the nerves in which it moves. His next job was to produce a vaccine as he had successfully done for anthrax. In that process, he had discovered the phenomenon of attenuation, of "weakening" of an infective agent by successive passages through various hosts.

He found that he could weaken the virus of rabies by passing it through a succession of animals and weaken it still further by drying the nervous tissue containing it before giving it to the next subject. Then he came to the decisive question, would injection of the weakened virus into an animal prevent it from acquiring rabies? He tried the experiment. Dogs were injected repeatedly with the weakened virus, each injection made stronger until he was satisfied that the animals could resist infection. Then he placed these dogs, protected by his series of injections, together with an equal number of untreated, unprotected dogs. A frantically mad dog was turned loose among the group. All were bitten. The unprotected dogs developed rabies; the ones vaccinated did not. Science at work.

Then Pasteur felt justified in announcing his method of protecting dogs against rabies; according to his ideas all dogs were to be inoculated and thus protected; rabies would then disappear as a disease of dogs and man for the most part. But there were difficulties in the way. There were stray dogs that could not be caught and protected, and there were wolves in France harboring rabies. Politicians and health officials got into the act. To them, Pasteur's approach was not practical. Matters were at an impasse.

Little Joseph Meister and his mother traveled from Alsace to Paris to go to Pasteur's laboratory to beg Pasteur to help them. The nine-year-old boy had been horribly bitten in fourteen places by a rabid dog. He was exposed to almost certain death. What could Pasteur do? Could he try his vaccine on the boy? Could he save Joseph's life? Could he prevent rabies? Or would this little boy die like thousands had before him?

Pasteur was not sure that he could do anything. His vaccine had been developed as a preventative measure for dogs, not a treatment for bitten children. He had never even planned to use it in that way. Prevention in animals is not the same as treatment in children.

Physicians were called in consultation, for Pasteur was a chemist, not a physician. They recommended that Pasteur make the attempt, since without it the boy was doomed. And so on July 16, 1885, at eight o'clock in the evening, sixty hours after the bite, the first injection was made. Each day thereafter until July 26th Joseph received injections of increasing strength. On that last day Pasteur did his supreme experiment. He injected the strongest concentration of rabies he could obtain—an injection that would kill an unprotected man. But little Joseph Meister was protected. The treatment had worked more rapidly than the virus from the bite of the dog could travel up his nerves. Rabies had been prevented. The boy survived.

Soon another patient appeared. Jean Baptiste Jupille, a shepherd boy who, seeing a mad dog throw itself upon a group of six young children, had taken his whip and rushed to their aid. The dog seized his hand. The boy threw the animal to the ground, forced open its mouth to release his mangled hand, and, although repeatedly bitten by the furious animal, he somehow held the dog while he tied its mouth shut with his whipcord and then beat it to death with his wooden shoe.

Jean Baptiste was treated by Pasteur. He was given the same series of shots that Joseph Meister had been given. Once again the method worked. The child did not develop rabies. And for eighty years, visitors to the Pasteur Institute could see a statue showing this shepherd boy struggling with the mad dog. It was more than a monument to his heroism; it marked the year when rabies was conquered. Science triumphant.

Telling the story like that, as it invariably is, leaves out a few details that might detract from its inherent romanticism. Today, we would not accept as proved that Joseph Meister or Jean Baptiste Jupille had actually been exposed to rabies. True, they had both been bitten by dogs, but not all dogs that bite nine-year-old boys or young shepherds are truly rabid; they do not all have rabies. Today, before giving anyone a course of vaccinations à la Pasteur to prevent rabies, every effort would be made to recover and study the brain of the dog. If the brain had evidence of rabies, the treatment would be initiated. If not, it would not.

Pasteur's experimental trials, of course, were based on the assumption that both dogs had rabies and the further assumption that the bite of a rabid dog always results in the transfer of the infection. But does it? Of course not. Virtually no infection has such 100 percent infectivity. Not tuberculosis. Not cholera. Not AIDS, and certainly not rabies. But it was always assumed that rabies did. It doesn't. How do we know? From episodes in which a single rabid animal attacked more than one person. The best-documented case took place some forty years ago in a small village in northern Iraq. A rabid animal attacked some three dozen people, biting them all, but only half got rabies. Why? We're not certain. One factor is obviously the variability in size of inoculum of live virus each of the victims received. That is how much virus was actually transferred. This in turn would depend upon a number of factors such as variability in amount of saliva and of concentration of virus in saliva. Other factors would also play a role, factors such as differences in the individual resistance of different people. All of these could be important.

Even if we assume that both dogs had rabies (two tacit,

unproven assumptions) the 50 percent infectivity sets up the following possibilities:

1) Neither of the two subjects had contracted rabies (25 percent).
2) One of the two subjects had contracted rabies (50 percent).
3) Both of the two subjects had contracted rabies (25 percent).

In short, no matter what, the fact that neither of the two patients died could well have been a random event and been unrelated to all of Pasteur's efforts. In fact, there is at least a 25 percent chance that that was true—assuming that both dogs had rabies.

One other factor is never included when this story is retold. What happened to the boys whose lives were saved? Joseph Meister became dedicated to Pasteur and the Pasteur Institute and remained there longer than the bronze statue of his fellow experimental subject. That statue, like many other such mementos in Paris, was melted down by the Germans during their occupation of Paris. At that time Joseph Meister was still working at the Pasteur Institute as concierge. And in that role, he collaborated with the Nazis. He told them who was Jewish, who had one Jewish parent, who was not loyal to the Germans, who could not be trusted, who came in at odd hours for clandestine meetings. So much for the little boy whose life was saved by one of the greatest names in the history of French science.

Or had Pasteur really saved his life?

Joseph Meister always believed that Pasteur saved him even while turning in Frenchmen who were hiding from the Nazis. Pasteur himself had far different feelings and loyalties. The Franco-Prussian war had been an unprovoked attack on France. The Germans, led by Prussia, united by Prussia, were not to be trusted. These feelings ran deep. Pasteur turned down the Prussian Cross of Merit. This great award, rarely given to non-Germans, was offered him for having developed the vaccine that saved Joseph Meister's life.

Hallervorden's Patients

The two victims I was reading about shared two extraordinarily unlikely aspects of their lives' stories. First, they both had the same inordinately rare neurologic disease; right now I cannot remember precisely which disease. It was one of those exceptionally uncommon hereditary degenerative disorders that begins in early childhood and leads inexorably to progressive loss of brain function. The degeneration results in loss of intellectual function, impairment and then loss of all motor function, and finally death. All this takes some eight to ten years while everyone stands by helplessly, unable to do much of anything. Of course, they died over half a century ago. Today, we can treat some of the causes of such deaths. We can treat the bacterial pneumonias with antibiotics so that the patients can live longer. Not exactly one of the triumphs of modern medicine.

Their disorder was genetic, a classic Mendelian recessive disease. In order for the brain to fall apart slowly over a decade or so, the child had to inherit one recessive gene from each parent. Those parents with one recessive gene and one normal dominant gene were, for all intents and purposes, normal. And they are, except that their children have a chance of getting the disease. What chance? A 25 percent chance. At meiosis, the father can produce two types of sperm: normal dominant sperm and abnormal recessive sperm, D and R. The same for the mother, D and R eggs. These can hook up randomly:

Sperm			Egg	
D	R		D	R
		Offspring		
DD		RD	DR	RR

So the odds for each child produced by the random coupling of one sperm from a father carrying the gene for the disease and one egg from a similar mother is this:

RR disease:	25%
DR or RD-carrier:	50%
DD-normal, neither disease nor carrier:	25%

Each child individually has a 25 percent chance of getting the disease and a 50 percent chance of being a carrier. But becoming a carrier doesn't cause much of a threat unless you marry another carrier, and carriers are rare, perhaps one in every fifteen or twenty thousand people. The odds are against procreating with another carrier unless, of course, you marry a first cousin descended from the same carrier grandparent. That changes the odds enormously.

The fact that the scientific paper I was reading described the pathologic finding in two patients with this, one of the rarest of all neurologic diseases, was not a coincidence or even unexpected. It was a paper by one of the well-known names in neuropathology, Hallervorden, and the disease in question was the subject of the paper. In it he described the gross pathology, what can be seen with the naked eye, as well as the microscopic pathology at two different stages of the disease. That was not unusual. Pneumonia strikes different patients at different times in the course of the disease. Nothing unusual about that.

And both patients died on the same day. Odd coincidence. Very unusual. As unlikely as marrying another random carrier. More than rare. Downright inexplicable!

How could that be? Two patients with the same rare affliction. Two patients who died in very different stages of disease. One died early in the course, he was only moderately disabled. The other died with severe disease, demented, immobile, bedridden. And they died on the same day. How could that be?

The date explained it all.

September 13, 1940. They had died on the same day and in the same place. In Nazi Germany. The cause of their deaths? I did not have to look. I knew. They had died as part of the program of euthanasia for various "defectives." In this program, institutionalized patients with any number of neurologic diseases were selected by SS physicians and then exterminated in a variety of prosaic, but labor-intensive ways, by other SS members. The methods varied from suffocation and strangulation, to carbon monoxide poisoning and . . . . The method did not matter. They all worked. So on September 13, 1940, these two patients became victims. They had not died; they had been murdered.

This program was started on September 1, 1939, on a direct order from Adolf Hitler. An organization was set up under the direction of Dr. Karl Brandt. State institutions were required to report all patients who had been ill five years or more and were unable to work. They had to fill out questionnaires giving name, race, marital status, nationality, next of kin, whether regularly visited and by whom, who bore financial responsibility, and so forth. The decision as to which patients should be killed was made entirely on the basis of this brief information and those fatal decisions were made by expert consultants. Most of these consultants never saw the patients themselves. They never examined them. They went over the sheets of information prepared by others. They reviewed this information and made a decision. Thumbs up or thumbs down. The thoroughness of those reviews can easily be evaluated. It can be reviewed far more thoroughly than the original review. One such "expert" working between November 14 and December 1, 1940, evaluated 2,109 questionnaires. Even if you assume that he worked every day (7 days a week), eight hours each day (no breaks), he would have spent less than three minutes scrutinizing each clinical evaluation. Three minutes to make each final decision. Not very much time, but perhaps it was "piecework."

These questionnaires were collected by a Realm's Work Committee of Institutions for Cure and Care. A parallel organization devoted exclusively to the killing of children was known by the similarly euphemistic name of Realm's Committee for Scientific Approach to Severe Illness Due to Heredity and Constitution. It was this organization which undoubtedly took care of these two children in a most scientific manner.

The Charitable Transport Company for the Sick then transported the chosen to the extermination centers. The Charitable Foundation for Institutional Care was then given the task of collecting the cost of the killings from the relatives of the poor deceased. Those relatives were never told precisely what the charges were for. And on the death certificates the cause of death was always falsified.

What these activities meant to the population at large was well expressed by those few hardy souls who dared to protest. A member of the court of appeals at Frankfurt am Main wrote in December, 1939:

> There is constant discussion of the question of the destruction of socially unfit life—in the places where there are mental institutions, in neighboring towns, sometimes over a large area, throughout the Rhineland, for example. The people have come to recognize the vehicles in which the patients are taken from their original institution to the intermediate institution and from there to the liquidation institution. I am told that when they see these buses even the children call out: "They're taking some more people to be gassed." From Limburg it is reported that every day from one to three buses with shades drawn pass through on the way from Weilmunster to Hadamar, delivering inmates to the liquidation institution there. According to the stories the arrivals are immediately stripped to the skin, dressed in paper shirts,

and forthwith taken to a gas chamber, where they are liquidated with hydrocyanic acid gas and an added anesthetic. The bodies are reported to be moved to a combustion chamber by means of a conveyor belt, six bodies to a furnace. The resulting ashes are then distributed into six urns which are shipped to the families. The heavy smoke from the crematory building is said to be visible over Hadamar every day. There is talk, furthermore, that in some cases heads and other portions of the body are removed for anatomical examination. The people working at this liquidation job in the institution, said to be assigned from other areas, are shunned completely by the populace. This personnel is described as frequenting the bars at night and drinking heavily. Quite apart from these overt incidents that exercise the imagination of the people, they are disquieted by the question of whether old folk who have worked hard all their lives and may merely have come into their dotage are also being liquidated. There is talk that the homes for the aged are to be cleaned out too. The people are said to be waiting for legislative regulation providing some orderly method that will insure especially that the aged feeble-minded are not included in the program.

Here one sees what "euthanasia" meant in actual practice. According to the records, 275,000 people were put to death in these killing centers. Ghastly as this seems, it should be realized that this program was merely the prelude for exterminations of far greater scope in the political program of genocide of conquered nations and the racially unwanted. The methods used and personnel trained in the killing centers for the chronically sick became the nucleus of the much larger centers in the East, where the plan was to kill all Jews and Poles and to cut down the Russian population by 30,000,000.

In Germany the exterminations included the mentally defective, psychotics (particularly schizophrenics), epileptics, and patients suffering from infirmities of old age and from various organic neurologic disorders such as infantile paralysis, Parkinsonism, multiple sclerosis, and brain tumors. The technical arrangements, methods, and training of the personnel who carried out the murders were under the direction of a committee of physicians and other experts headed by Dr. Karl Brandt. The mass killings were the first carried out with carbon monoxide gas, but later cyanide gas ("cyclon B") was found to be more efficient. The idea of camouflaging the gas chambers as shower baths was developed by Brandt, who testified in court that the patients walked in calmly, deposited their towels and stood with their little pieces of soap under the shower outlets waiting for the water to start running. All those unable to work and considered non-rehabilitable were killed.

Dr. Hallervorden obtained hundreds of brains from the killing centers for the insane. He himself gave a vivid firsthand account of his activity. The Charitable Transport Company for the Sick brought the brains in batches of 150 to 250 at a time. Hallervorden stated:

> There was wonderful material among those brains, beautiful mental defectives, malformations and early infantile diseases. I accepted those brains of course. Where they came from and how they came to me was really none of my business.

In addition to the material he wanted, all kinds of other cases were mixed in, such as patients suffering from various types of parkinsonism, simple depressions, involutional depressions and brain tumors, and all kinds of other illnesses, including psychopathy that had been difficult to handle:

> These were selected from the various wards of the institutions according to an excessively simple and quick method. Most institutions did not have enough physicians, and what physicians there were were either too busy or did not care, and they delegated the selection to the nurses and attendants. Whoever looked sick or was otherwise a problem was put on a list and was transported to the killing center. The worst thing about this business was that it produced a certain brutalization of the nursing personnel. They got to simply picking out those whom they did not like, and the doctors had so many patients that they did not even know them, and put their names on the list.

Of the patients thus killed, only the brains were sent to Dr. Hallervorden; they were killed in such large numbers that autopsies of the bodies were not feasible. That, in Dr. Hallervorden's opinion, greatly reduced the scientific value of the material. The brains, however, were always well fixed and suspended in formalin, exactly according to his own instructions.

Hallervorden should have known better. He never understood how wrong he had been. After the war was over, he admitted that the entire field of German psychiatry had been permanently hurt by the activities of the euthanasia program and that psychiatrists had lost the respect of the German people forever. Dr. Hallervorden concluded: "Still, there were interesting cases in this material."

It is as if the German people were ready to accept the exterminations of the sick far more readily than they were to accept murder for political reasons. Perhaps that is why initial exterminations of the political opponents were carried out under the guise of psychiatric sickness. So-called psychiatric experts were dispatched to survey the inmates of camps with the specific order to pick out members of racial minorities and political offenders from occupied territories and to dispatch them to the extermination centers with specially created psychiatric diagnoses such as "inveterate German-hater." This diagnosis was frequently given to prisoners who had been active in the Czech underground. Only a psychiatric disorder could account for such behavior.

Certain classes of patients with mental diseases who were considered to be able to perform labor, particularly members of the armed forces suffering from psychopathy or neurosis, were sent to concentration camps to be worked to death or were reassigned to punishment battalions and were exterminated in the process of removing of minefields by stepping on mines.

A large number of those marked for death for political or racial reasons were made available for "medical" experiments involving the use of involuntary human subjects. From 1942 on, such experiments which had been carried out in concentration camps were openly presented at German medical meetings. This program included "terminal human experiments," a term that denoted an experiment so designed that its successful conclusion depended on the test subject being put to death. A clear end point.

And after the war, after his admissions quoted above, Hallervorden submitted a paper to be presented at the first postwar Congress of Neuropathology. Its subject was "The Neuropathology of Mental Defectives in the Nazi Euthanasia Program." It was not the study of the brains that was wrong, only the bad reputation of the program itself.

The paper was rejected. The world did not accept Hallervorden's hypothesis that how the brain came to be in his possession made no difference:

> There was wonderful material among those brains, beautiful mental defectives, malformations and early infantile diseases. I accepted those brains of course. Where they came from and how they came to me was really none of my business.

20

EL CID IN THE OFFICE

A doctor's reputation is made by the number of great men who die under his care.

George Bernard Shaw

Names are not my forte. They never have been and they never will be. Among my students and colleagues, my inability to recall names is legendary. It may be one of the reasons I am so understanding of my older patients with their benign, and at times not so benign, memory loss of aging.

My poor ability to remember names plagues me both personally and professionally every day of my life. So I play a game with myself, a game of associations. I associate the name of the patient with a name I already know. Old baseball players. Especially the names of old Chicago White Sox players so indelibly etched into my memory. I also use the names of authors, writers of every description, and historical figures.

In this way, Mrs. Barbara Nicholson, a woman with Parkinson's disease whom I first saw in 1971, became "Big Swish." "Big Swish" Nicholson had been a slugging outfielder for the Chicago Cubs of my youth. Her doctor said that levodopa wasn't for her. It was too risky. She didn't believe that; she'd heard about patients who had been helped by it. She came to see me. I put her on levodopa and she responded. "Big Swish" remained my patient for a decade.

Other patients acquired such new names as William Faulkner (real name Elizabeth), T. S. (James) Eliot, Karel Vapek, P. G. Wodehouse, Eugene O'Neill, Tennessee Williams, Ezra Pound, and Alfonso Rodrigo.

As soon as I saw the name *Rodrigo* on the chart, I made the necessary associations and labeled the patient Alfonso, although on all the forms the name was José A. Rodrigo.

Alfonso Rodrigo. The titles of his books, I've never forgotten. The *Dreams of Don Quixote, El Cid on 22nd Street.* After Saul Bellow, he was Chicago's best-known resident author. More than that, he was one of the great Latin writers.

Alfonso Rodrigo. I thought to myself as I called out the last name Rodrigo and scanned the room.

A man who looked to be about sixty got up.

"This will be easy," I said to myself. He looks like my image of Alfonso Rodrigo. Short but sturdy.

Long graying hair. More a mane than just hair. A perfect frame for his face. Craggy, chiseled, weathered. With a glint in his bright black eyes. It was the face I would always associate with the name. Here was El Cid reborn. Here was a man who was closer to El Cid than whatever actor had played the role in the Hollywood version of *El Cid on 22nd Street*. Remembering this man's name would be easier than "Big Swish" Nicholson, or "Swede" Risberg.

Alfonso Rodrigo, né José, walked toward me. He moved his arms normally. As he stepped forward with his right leg, his right arm swung backwards and his left arm swung forward, smoothly, freely. When his left leg moved forward, the arms changed positions ever so smoothly. No decreased arm swing on either side. To me that meant that Al (I knew that he liked to be called Al) didn't have Parkinson's disease. I observed that his right leg moved normally, but his left didn't. He raised his left knee higher than normal, as if he were raising his left foot to step up onto a curb, but his left foot didn't lift. The heel came off the ground, but the toes didn't. And then he repeated the same process. His right leg moved normally. His left didn't.

"A drop foot on the left," I diagnosed quietly to myself. Most likely due to some sort of injury to a nerve called the peroneal nerve which controls those muscles that lift the toes off the ground.

I led Al Rodrigo into the examining room and we both sat down and I introduced myself. "What," I asked, "brings you to see me?"

"I want you to answer a simple question for me," he said.

His voice was strong, rich, the perfect voice for the real Alfonso Rodrigo.

"And what is that?" I inquired.

He stared at me. His eyes penetrated me, his voice shook, ever so slightly. "How long do I have to live?"

"How long . . . ." I echoed. This man seemed to exude life, to exemplify living, yet he already knew he was dying and had just one question. Not about his diagnosis. Not about his treatment. About his prognosis.

210

"How long," he repeated with slightly more of a quiver this time, "do I have to live?"

Over the next hour I teased out his entire medical history. He was fifty-eight years old. He had been born and raised in Chicago, although he now lived in Indiana. He had been in good health until some six months before, when suddenly he began to have trouble with his left foot.

What kind of trouble?

It dragged. He couldn't lift it.

What had he meant by suddenly?

One night he went to bed a normal man, the next morning he awoke a dying man.

I needed facts, not such self-indulgent musings. In the end I got them, bit by bit. Each bit associated with cosmic considerations on life and death, the meaning of that reality, the reality of that meaning.

This man Rodrigo had been in perfect health. Then, he has a sudden foot drop on the left. It had started acutely and there had been no progression. An acute drop foot like his usually was not a death sentence. It was rarely the first manifestation of a fatal illness. Usually it was due to external pressure on the peroneal nerve as it passed behind the knee joint. It often signified a mild degree of inflammation or disease of the nerves in general, a peripheral neuropathy or neuritis, but that type of condition is only rarely the sign of a rapidly progressing fatal disease.

What other symptoms did he have?

His list was as inexhaustible as that magnificent voice of his.

And it began with his voice. It was not what it had once been.

I had all I could do not to laugh out loud. There was nothing wrong with the voice I had been listening to.

He was losing his voice. It was all but destroyed already. The projection was gone. The inflections. The timbre. The quality. And that voice was his life. He, like his voice, was dying. It had been a gift from God. And now God was withdrawing that gift inch by inch, decibel by decibel.

How long before he became a monotone? Then mute? Silenced? Unable to speak?

How long?

He was already monotonous. Except there was a better medical term for it. He was obsessed. Not with life. Not even with death. But with coming to terms with death, doing battle with his own mortality. His other symptoms were all as poignant as his speech problems. Each threatened his life. Each typified his impending death.

No doctors were allowed to partake in that battle. Our role was merely to observe, to document the wounds, and tell one combatant how many rounds he had left.

I examined him.

He had a foot drop on the left. And nothing else. Absolutely nothing else.

Had he seen any other neurologists?

He had.

What had they told him?

That he was dying.

Of what?

Lou Gehrig's disease. Amyotrophic lateral sclerosis.

He must have seen the disbelief that wrinkled my forehead.

"I have their records. And the EMGs. Right here." He reached into his pocket and gave them to me. "Read these," he said, with the fervor of an apostle handing the Gospels to an unconverted heathen.

I devoured the reports word for word. No one had ever been more willing to be converted. But to what?

There was no hard evidence that he had ALS, no real facts supporting that diagnosis. The neurologists—some of the most respected in Chicago—had found nothing. Just this man and his unending litany of his vision of his own decay and death. And they bought it, hook, line, and sinker. Lou Gehrig's disease. Amyotrophic lateral sclerosis, ALS. And with that diagnosis came death.

How soon?

A year, two. Perhaps three. If he were lucky.

I was not so easily sold. I remained unconverted.

I told him he did not have ALS. He was not dying. He had a mild neuropathy. No big deal. Life would go on. His voice was not threatened, that voice on which he depended for his livelihood.

By the way, I asked, "What do you do for a living?"

"I am a writer," he said.

A writer.

He was not just any Alfonso Rodrigo, but El Cid of Iberian legend.

I saw him as a patient for a few more times. Each visit was the same. He told me of his symptoms, those impediments God had inflicted upon him as a sign of His power and Alfonso Rodrigo's impotence.

Each time I examined him and found nothing.

No weakness.

All he had was a foot drop that was getting better.

Each time I told him he was not dying. And each time he looked at me sadly with the look of someone misunderstood.

Five visits were enough. He was getting better. I could not help him and I was bored by his game. I said goodbye and sent him out without scheduling another visit. He could fight his battle in front of a different witness.

I next saw Alfonso Rodrigo five years later. He was doing a public reading of a couple of his short stories. I sat in the back of the room and watched him walk up to the stage. The foot drop was gone. His hair was longer, whiter, making a longer, richer mane. Moses in the wilderness.

And his voice had not changed at all. It had lost none of its timbre, none of its force, its inflections, its richness.

The stories were him. Latinos from the South Side of Chicago meeting their fates, coming to terms with life and death.

As he walked out, he spied me.

I nodded.

He stared.

This time it was his face that was mistrustful, not mine.

I started to call his name.

The mistrust turned into something far more angry.

I stopped.

He walked on by with no sign of any foot drop.

Lou Gehrig had only lived two years once his ALS took hold. None of his symptoms ever got better.

Three years after that last interaction, I was forced to recall the entire episode. My wife and I had gone out to dinner with another Chicago area writer, William Brashler, and his wife Cindy.

They had been with the Rodrigos the previous weekend. Bill had mentioned my name to Al. Al had become livid. I represented all that was wrong with medicine in the United States. He ranted and raved about how terrible I was.

Bill wanted to know what had happened. Was I all that bad? He'd thought I was supposed to be a good neurologist.

Cindy was even more curious.

What could I say? Since Alfonso Rodrigo had been my patient, my professional interactions with him were confidential.

They were both persistent.

It was my wife who came to the rescue.

She knew Al. The Rodrigos lived in Indiana, not far from where she had grown up. Her folks knew the Rodrigos. In fact, her mom's best friend was their next-door neighbor.

Barbara skillfully shifted the conversation away from me and my confrontation with Alfonso Rodrigo. She told a story her parents had told her. It had taken place ten years earlier. Her parents had been invited to the Rodrigos for dinner. Her dad's an ophthalmologist. Al had been intrigued by that fact. Al had trouble with his eyes. Serious trouble. Progressive trouble. He was, in fact, going blind.

A blind writer. He would no longer be able to see his words on the page, to feel the flow. He was doomed, like Beethoven. Worse, like Henri Matisse, who could no longer hold a paint brush.

There was not a dry eye in the house.

Barb's dad asked the diagnosis.

"Retinitis pigmentosa."

Were the doctors certain?

Al shrugged. Were they ever?

Another opinion couldn't hurt.

Al agreed.

Barb's mom and dad left, much saddened by the tragedy that they now knew was plaguing Alfonso Rodrigo. Poor Al, fighting against certain blindness. Perhaps there was something Barb's dad could do to help him.

Al never came to see Barb's dad. He never made an appointment.

"But his vision is fine," Bill said.

"He reads without glasses," Cindy added.

I merely laughed. Again I had to face their questions.

I said the only thing I could. "He wanted me to witness his struggle with mortality."

"That's Al," Bill said. "That's what he asks of us all."

"True," I said. "But I refused to participate. As a friend I could have, but not as a professional."

21

A Trip to Vienna

Of people I knew who are now in the serious dirt of the ditches at Dachau.

John Stone, MD
Looking Down into a Ditch

In late 1989, I was invited to act as co-chairman at a festive meeting to be held in Vienna in honor of Walter Birkmayer's eightieth birthday. I felt quite honored by the invitation. Birkmayer had done more for Parkinson's disease than any other clinician. He deserved to be honored. There have been only three major clinical discoveries made in our field in the last thirty years and Birkmayer made them all. The first was that levodopa worked, that it made Parkinson's disease better. The second was that giving levodopa, in combination with another molecule, changed how the body metabolized levodopa, made the levodopa safer, easier on the patient and more effective. And the third and most recent, was that an entirely different medication, deprenyl, changed the natural history of the disease itself and allowed patients with Parkinson's disease to live longer. Birkmayer deserved a gala affair and I was honored to act as co-chairman.

They would pay my and my wife's way, of course, and all of our expenses. The timing was perfect. The meeting was to be held in Vienna on May 15, 1990. Spring in Vienna and then we'd go to London. My British publisher wanted me to be in London around that time for the publication of my next book, *Newton's Madness*. We both loved London and my wife had never been to Vienna.

As always, the thought of being in Vienna was not entirely pleasant for me. I know that for many people Vienna brings forth pleasant associations: the music of the Strauss family, waltzes, Sachertorte, coffee shops, schlag, strolls along the Ringstrasse, color, light.

But for me, Vienna was a city of brilliance and tragedy, of genius and repression, of culture and hatred. The city where in just a few brief decades Schönberg and his students, Berg and Webern, reshaped the structure of music. Schönberg was eventually driven out, since he had been born Jewish. Webern stayed and was shot by a GI shortly after World War II, wandering on the Ringstrasse in the rubble of the Opera House. Vienna had always been the heart of the anti-Semitism that pervaded the official life of the Austro-Hungarian empire. The Vienna where Mahler was forced to convert to become the conductor of the State Opera. Where Freud never got a professorship. Where Karposi who described Karposi's sarcoma converted and changed his name from Cohen to Karposi in order to get a job. A city that had convinced the world that Hitler was a German and Beethoven an Austrian. Vienna was not to be trusted.

The last time I had been there, with my son, our visit had coincided with a visit by the Pope. He had then gone to the local concentration camp, Matthausen, and talked about all of the suffering of the victims and how they should not be forgotten, and not once mentioned the word *Jew*.

However, I also had positive associations with Vienna, especially the Vienna of Birkmayer. I spent several days there in 1971 as Birkmayer's guest. He personally showed me his laboratories and his clinical research facility. We strolled together on the Ringstrasse talking about Parkinson's disease. He had others in his department drive me around town. I was his colleague, his compatriot. They were all kind, friendly.

Everyone in Vienna told me their stories. The Jews they had helped, the risks they had taken, the souls they had saved. I left feeling much like the great pianist Arthur Rubenstein. A reporter from *Time* magazine had once asked Rubenstein why he never played in Germany, the land of Beethoven.

"It wouldn't be fair to the ninety million Jews of West Germany," Rubenstein replied.

"But there aren't ninety million Jews in West Germany," the reporter countered naively.

"There must be," the pianist objected. "After all, there are thirty million West Germans, and each one I ever met personally saved three Jews during the War."

Two weeks before I was to leave for Vienna for the Birkmayer celebration, I was at the office of the United Parkinson Foundation. The Chicago based UPF is one of the major not-for-profit groups that supports research and patient services in Parkinson's disease. I'm chairman of its Medical Advisory Board. It occurred to me that the executive director of the UPF, Judy Rosner, might have some pictures of Walter Birkmayer at past meetings or other such memorabilia, and as chairman of the opening session, I could humanize the program a bit by slipping these in as I reminisced about Birkmayer's accomplishments.

Judy looked through her files and found several good pictures of Birkmayer waltzing in Vienna.

"Perhaps," I added half-jokingly, "we could even find a picture of Birkmayer in his old SS uniform."

She gave me a puzzled look. I explained that I had long ago heard two vague rumors about Birkmayer. The first was he had been a doctor in the SS, the second that he was part Jewish. "I always said both were probably true," I said. There had, I knew, been a Birkmayer who had converted to become director of the ballet corps at the Opera during the late nineteenth century. Perhaps that Birkmayer was related in some way to our Birkmayer.

I tried to make light of it. Perhaps Birkmayer, I suggested, had Waldheim's disease, the new neurologic disorder names after the president of Austria. It was a variant of Alzheimer's disease. While in Alzheimer's all memory is lost, in Waldheim's disease, there is a much more circumscribed memory loss—a peculiar inability to remember being a Nazi.

Neither of us laughed.

Rumors were no longer sufficient. I needed facts; I had to know one way or the other. The rumors, I was certain, had to be just rumors. Idle gossip. Birkmayer befriended me yet he knew I was Jewish. And I wasn't the only Jew he'd been associated with over the years. There were others who were a lot closer to him, who worked with him, collaborated with him. One of them lived in Israel and yet worked in Birkmayer's laboratory for several months each year. They had to have checked him out. Still, I had to know. Conjecture was not sufficient if I was to honor this man.

I called the Simon Weisenthal Center. If anyone had the facts, it would be the people there. The telephone receptionist connected me with a member of their research department. I asked him about Birkmayer.

"I have the file right here," he began.

A file. Right there. I felt chilly.

"His SS number was 309 088."

He read me the details from the file. One at a time. Birkmayer had been an SS physician. He had not just been a Nazi, he'd been in the SS. Birkmayer had been a Unterstürmführer or second lieutenant. Birkmayer had, of course, volunteered to serve in the SS. All SS members were volunteers. This was not the army. It was the SS. Serving in the army was no crime. You got drafted; you went. You did your duty. What choice did you have? But Birkmayer had not waited to be drafted. He'd volunteered for the SS!

He accepted his commission on September 11, 1938. His Nazi party number was 612 6594. He had joined the party in May 1938. He had been dismissed from the SS on December 21, 1939, when it was discovered that, unbeknownst to Birkmayer, he was not a pure Aryan.

My God! Both rumors were true! He was part Jewish and he had been a physician in the SS. Why hadn't I checked before? Why hadn't anyone else? "To be in the SS, a person had to be proven to have no Jewish blood back to 1800. To be an officer, that date was moved back to 1750," my contact informed me. "All SS officers were volunteers. They had to pass three tests: a physical examination, an ideological examination, and then a racial background search. In the long run, Birkmayer flunked number three." But he had passed the ideological exam. He was voluntarily an officer of an outlaw organization. It was because of the ideological purity that Hitler trusted the SS. He didn't trust the army. They were not ideologically pure. "Members of the SS pledged their loyalty to Hitler himself."

"What's that?" I asked.

"SS members had only one loyalty. Not to Germany. Not to the Third Reich. But to Der Führer."

My head was spinning. Birkmayer. SS and SS physician. A Nazi doctor. Loyalty to Der Führer. Racial purity. I could not believe my ears.

"When he was dismissed, Birkmayer received a letter commending him on his services to the SS. That letter was signed on behalf of Adolf Hitler."

"My God."

"Of course, it may not be the same Birkmayer. Mine's a neurologist."

So's mine, I thought.

"The best way to be certain," he said, "is to check the birth date. This Birkmayer was born on . . . ."

"May 15, 1910," I interrupted him.

"Yes," he said. "He'll be eighty in . . . ."

"Two weeks," I said. I knew his birthdate. That was the date of the meeting I was supposed to chair. "He was born on May 10, 1910."

"That's the date. That's the right Birkmayer."

He was wrong. It was the wrong Birkmayer. The most wrong Birkmayer it could be.

We talked for another ten minutes. I don't recall anything else that either of us said, except that he promised to send me a copy of all the documents. I'd already heard too much that I could never forget.

This was a man with whom I had broken bread more than once, over two decades.

"Did Rubenstein ever play in Vienna?" I mused aloud.

I could not go to Vienna. I could not co-chair the meeting. I sent off a fax to the organizers of the meeting, telling them that because of Professor Birkmayer's professional activities in 1938 and 1939, I could not participate in any festivities honoring his lifetime accomplishments.

Was I the first to have that knowledge? Had others known? Had they come to terms with it differently than I had? Had they kept Birkmayer's little secret?

Why couldn't I? Because it wouldn't have been fair to the ninety million Jews of West Germany.

The documents came and with them knowledge. As long as Birkmayer's Nazi proclivities were a rumor, the implications could be ignored. His name and birthdate on a list of SS appointments dated 1 December 1938 changed that irrevocably.

Abram	Karl	309087	8.03.09
Dr. Birkmayer	Walter	309088	15.05.10
Braun	Gustav	309089	21.06.90
Brunner	Helmut	309090	16.09.13

What had been conjecture was now irrefutable fact. This called for some sort of response, some kind of activity. It could not just sit there as a fact, cold, isolated, removed from my life, insulated from my thoughts, quarantined from my behavior. It pervaded everything.

I could not go to Vienna.

But what of the others? My professional colleagues who had also been invited to honor Unterstürmführer Birkmayer. Some were Jews, from the United States, England, Israel. And some of them were my friends. Should they be told? Did I have the right to complicate their lives, to force them to share the same burden? Did I have the right not to? Wasn't it an obligation, not a right? Has it not been Elie Wiesel's message that survivors had to be witnesses? Did that not also mean that all others who knew significant facts could also not remain silent?

The next day I went to Washington for the first International Congress of the Movement Disorder Society (a scientific club of all of us who have dedicated our careers to studying movement disorders, such as Parkinson's disease). All of my professional friends were there. Many of them were going to Vienna. The first person I saw was Joe Jankovic, a movement-disorder specialist in Houston. His name was on the program for the Birkmayer gala celebration. He told me that he and his wife were going to Vienna. They had tickets to the Staatsoper to see Mozart, that had cost $150 each. Joe was the son of survivors. He'd been born in Czechoslovakia.

I told him what I knew.

"When I was a kid in high school, I belonged to the Young Communist Club."

"Birkmayer was twenty-eight," I said.

"Do you know anyone who likes Mozart?" he replied, "I have two extra tickets to *Giovanni*. It's a great production."

Next came Stan Fahn, one of the most respected of all movement-disorder specialists. We had been trying to set a date for a future meeting, not an easy task considering our busy schedules.

"May fifteenth," I suggested.

"Vienna," he protested.

I told him what I knew.

"May fifteen it is," he said.

Then the furor began. Everyone heard bits and pieces of the story and came to me for verification. One of those was Peter Riederer, a neuroscientist from Vienna whom I knew and respected. Peter was too young to have been involved. He had worked with Birkmayer. He'd known him for years. I told Peter what I knew.

"I must call Birkmayer," he said. "There must be a mistake here. He'll straighten it out."

Peter called Vienna. It was the first of a series of such calls.

"Birkmayer denies ever having been in the SS," he told me.

I showed him the documents. He read them, once, twice. He stared at the list of members for a full fifteen minutes.

"I must call him again," he mumbled. "He is getting old; his memory, perhaps—"

"Waldheim's disease," I replied.

Peter did not understand. I did not take the time to explain.

He made his second call and then sought me out once again.

"He was only in the SS for a couple of months, He never left Vienna."

"Years," I said pointing out the dates.

Another call.

"He was on the Russian front the entire time." As if being on the Russian front absolved him of all taint. Had there been no Babi Yar?

Birkmayer on the Russian front!

In 1938.

What had he been, a lonely advance scout?

"There was no Russian front in 1938. Just the home front," I reminded him. He had to know the dates as well as I did.

It went on and on. Finally, Birkmayer said if we would come to Vienna, he would make a public statement clearing it all up. He would come clean.

No Americans went to the meeting. Many Europeans did, as did two Israelis with long, complicated ties to Vienna and Birkmayer. The Israelis had been promised that the statement would explain everything.

There was no statement. Not a word was said except to deplore the actions of that man from Chicago who accused Birkmayer of committing war crimes. I never made such an accusation. I do not know what he did specifically. I do not want to know. But I do know one thing—that if no one had volunteered for the SS, the Holocaust might have been very different.

My wife and I did go to London. And my publisher hosted a luncheon for us and our British friends. One of those was a neurologist who had gone to Vienna. I had called him from Washington. I had told him the entire story.

"What did he do?" he had asked.

"He was in the SS."

"What specifically?"

"He joined the SS."

"Did he commit any war crimes?"

"I have no idea. But when he was discharged, the notice of his dismissal went to the Sanitary Bureau."

"The Sanitary Bureau. That sounds innocent enough."

"They ran the euthanasia program."

He went to Vienna. Why? Birkmayer had promised to tell all.
And he confided in me: "Birkmayer said nothing."
What had he really expected?

This story has no ending. The Ninth International Parkinson's
Disease Congress was held in Japan in October 1991. The Honorary
Chairman was Walter Birkmayer. I was invited to participate, to give
a paper on brain implants. I could not honor this man. So I stayed
home.

For me it was an easy although not ambivalent decision. For
others it was not easy. The organizers could not understand my position and demanded that I explain fully why I was acting as I was. The
organizers then wrote to other participants trying to assure their participation and enclosing a letter from Birkmayer in which he wrote
that if anyone could find "*one* Jewish man" to whom he had done any
harm, he would pay one million Austrian schillings to a Jewish char-
ity in Vienna. The responses varied. Copies of many were sent to me,
as an apparently interested party. Two came from Israeli neurologists, both close friends of mine. The first wrote:

> Prof. Birkmayer joined a criminal organization with the ideology
> of genocide against the Jewish people. In his letter to Melvin Yahr, Prof.
> Birkmayer neither expresses any regret nor shows any sensitivity. I
> found his letter insulting, and I will refrain from commenting on his offer
> "to pay one million schilling." The Nazi leader of Germany during those
> years also did not personally "harm" any Jew, but his organization,
> where Prof. Birkmayer was a member, was responsible for all the atroc-
> ities that were committed against the Jews. A person such as Prof.
> Birkmayer should be probably reprimanded as a war criminal and not
> be excused by Jewish people. We are not to forgive him on behalf of the
> people against whom his organization committed those crimes.

The second wrote this:

> I can appreciate the difficult times you are having with the
> Birkmayer affair. I have no sympathy for Dr. Birkmayer. His old age of
> 80 years and the distance from the terrible Nazi period, do not make
> the situation any better or forgivable. His explanatory statement which
> I have now seen for the first time, is so revolting and disgusting to me
> that I find it difficult to understand why you are spreading it around. I
> cannot give you or him my understanding. I definitely do not and never
> did want any more explanations from him. A large part of my family per-
> ished in Europe fifty years ago and I (already and luckily born in Israel)
> was brought up on their memories.

To me, this affair is entirely dissociated from the Parkinson's Disease meeting and I am attending the Conference anyway. It is too important for me to skip it for this Birkmayer. I think it was distasteful in the first place to give him the honor, but I tend to agree with you that it may be too late now to change the decision.

Everyone emotionally involved will make his own judgement and decision about attending . . . .

PART FIVE

LIFE, DEATH, AND IN BETWEEN

We know the mathematical equations that govern normal matter, but we cannot solve them exactly except in very simple situations. Even a problem as simple as that of three bodies interacting under the Newtonian law of gravity can be solved only approximately. Yet the human body contains about a thousand mission million million million particles (one with twenty-seven zeros).

Stephen Hawking
"The Unification of Physics"

All the King's horses
And all the King's men
Couldn't put Humpty
Together again.

Mother Goose's Melody

22

COMING IN FIRST

"Shut up," he explained.

Ring Lardner

Millions long for immortality who don't know what to do with themselves on a rainy Sunday afternoon.

Susan Ertz

It was the late sixties and the race was on. Not the arms race. Not the race to put the first man on the moon; that had already been won. This was a far more important race—for the administration of our hospital. It was a race for fame, stature, notoriety, and with those, new patients. For that's the bottom line, attracting patients and keeping the beds filled. It came down to the race to become the first medical center in Chicago to perform a heart transplant.

And that first would come with all the trappings: TV news, newspapers, word of mouth. All resulting in our becoming synonymous with heart surgery in the hearts and minds of physicians all over the Midwest, physicians who just might have patients who needed to have heart surgery and had to be referred somewhere.

But that's what show business is all about. The fact that we had no transplant specialists in our institution didn't seem to matter. We had done no kidney transplants. We had lots of kidney specialists. We did dialysis, but not transplants. These we referred elsewhere. Why? Because we had no transplant surgeons. And we had no one with any experience in the chronic immune suppression that such patients require. So what? We had cardiac surgeons and patients. And there were more patients out there. So many more, all looking for the best cardiac surgery program in town. For the first team that did a transplant.

All we needed was a donor.

Before anyone else got one.

The word went out across the entire state. Needed: one cardiac donor. A patient who had been in good health and had gotten himself killed, suddenly, in some sort of accident. That happened every day.

But a patient killed in a particular way. A way in which the brain died but the heart went on.

We got one.

That was how I became involved. It was my job as the neurologist to make sure that the donor was dead, or at least that his brain was dead. For death had suddenly ceased to be a simple question. I was asked by my chairman to be on call to come into the hospital any time of the day or night to certify that the donor's brain was dead.

"Whose decision will that be?" I asked, not wanting to examine the patient/donor with a team of anxious surgeons breathing down my neck.

"Yours."

"Mine alone?" I asked.

"Yes."

That was one step in the right direction. That meant that the cardiovascular surgeons would have no say. And they shouldn't. They could not exactly be impartial.

"What criteria do I use?"

"Yours. The usual ones. Whatever you think is appropriate."

"I think it would be appropriate if we stayed out of this business altogether."

"That is not one of your options," I was told.

I nodded. I understood precisely what was wanted.

The criteria for brain death are not that complicated. They all break down to the absence of all brain activity over a given period of time. But there are three catches. How to you prove the brain isn't working? How can you be certain that its inactivity is irreversible? And for how long?

Neurologists all know what to test, those basic, primitive functions housed in the brain stem. There are only a few things to check. It takes less that five minutes.

Is there any movement? Either spontaneously or in response to pain?

Is there any ventilation? For it is nothing more than a movement.

Do the pupils react to light?

Do the eyes move? Spontaneously? In response to a strong stimulus? To the strongest? That's tested by running ice-cold water into the ear. The ice water stimulates the inner ear to cause eye movement. This is the maximal stimulus that can be given to the brain stem.

And an electroencephalogram, an EEG. The brain waves must be flat.

I was all set. Optimist that I am.

The first phone call came at about eleven-thirty on a Thursday night. The donor had been found. In Peoria. He was twenty-five and had driven his car into a tree. He'd been pronounced dead at the scene of the accident.

"Had he been drinking?" I asked.

"What difference does that make?" the cardiac surgeon responded.

"If his blood alcohol level is too high, I can't pronounce him brain dead. Some of the loss of activity could be due to the alcohol." And, I added to myself, most young drivers who run into trees have been drinking.

"Don't be obstructive," he added, clarifying the situation. "We're making arrangements to fly him to Chicago."

"A Medevac ambulance?"

"No, a private plane. A Cessna. He doesn't need much care. Someone will ventilate him with an ambu set-up."

An ambu is a hand-operated ventilator. Rather like the bladder of a football, it's attached to a tube placed into the patient's trachea. The operator ventilates the patient by compressing the large air-filled rubber bladder, thus pushing air or oxygen into the lungs.

They would pack the donor into a four-seat Cessna and bounce him to Chicago, ambuing him all the way. They hoped he'd arrive around two. They were calling in the recipient and hoped to have his chest opened by four. They'd call back when they needed me—in a couple of hours.

I got to the hospital a little after two in the morning. Tom Benton was in the Surgical Intensive Care Unit. He was a farm boy from Iowa. Martin Lewis, the potential recipient, was also in the SICU, in a different room, being prepared for the surgery.

The cardiac surgeon greeted me. "No alcohol. Never drinks. Against his religion. Or something. No drugs. You can check with his

229

fiancée. She's at his bedside.

I did not have to ask which patient was which. One end of the ICU was a bustle of activity. Four cardiovascular surgeons, the entire corporation. Three cardiovascular surgery fellows, residents, nurses, techs, hospital administrators. Even someone from public relations, and the Vice President for Philanthropy.

At the other end of ICU, things were a bit quieter.

One patient.

One ventilator going whoosh-whoosh. The ambu bag had been replaced by a full-fledged ventilator.

One lone technician, attaching electrodes to Tom Benton's head.

And one very bewildered young woman in a dress that was forty years out of style, as if she had walked out of a Grant Wood painting and into the twenty-first century.

I walked over to her side and introduced myself. I did not tell her what my role was. There seemed to be no reason to add to her grief or bewilderment. Her Tom was already dead. She had flown up here in that same plane while the local doctor had pushed air in and out of Tom's dead body.

"I'm a neurologist," I began. I had to tell her something.

She said nothing. We stood side by side watching the ventilator and the EEG technician.

I told her what the EEG tech was doing.

Still she said nothing.

All that greeted my words was the continuous whooshing of the ventilator. Whoosh . . . whoosh.

I told her what I had to do.

She said nothing.

Whoosh . . . whoosh.

I told her what I would be testing. Pain response. Pupillary response to light. Ice water into his ears.

She said nothing. She never even looked at me. Her eyes were glued on Tom.

Whoosh . . . whoosh.

I went on and on.

It was as if she didn't hear me, as if I did not exist. Her world consisted of her and Tom and the ventilator. And soon that would be turned off and she would be all alone.

When I got to the front of the bed, the EEG tech smiled at me. I took out my flashlight and started to open Tom Benton's eyes.

"She's deaf," the tech said.

I stopped.

"Who's deaf?" I asked quietly, afraid of what I would hear.

"The fiancée," I was told.

It was like I had stepped into a scene from a Woody Allen movie. "How about the patient?" I asked.

The tech shrugged.

I turned to the fiancée. "I'm Dr. Klawans," I began.

She nodded ever so slightly.

"I'm a neurologist."

She smiled faintly.

"I'm going to examine Tom."

"Yes," she said in a peculiarly pitched, hardly modulated voice.

"You read lips?"

She nodded.

No more beating around the bush.

"Was Tom deaf?"

"Yes."

That was what I had feared.

I flashed the light in his right eye.

It reacted. The pupil immediately contracted down.

Normally.

I flashed the light into his left eye.

It too, reacted. Normally.

His brain stem was working.

Tom was not brain dead.

Far from it. His brain stem was working.

Normally.

I turned back to his fiancée. I asked her her name.

Ever-good," she said, as if the syllables were each independent words. "Fran-ces Ever-good."

"Frances," I asked, "does Tom read lips?" I hoped she did not notice my change in tenses.

"Yes," she said. Even I could tell from her tone and her entire being she had noticed.

Tom's eyes were still open. The lids had not fallen into a closed position. They were being held open by Tom's own efforts.

I moved until my face was above his eyes.

"Tom," I began.

His eyes opened wider.

He was awake and alert.

231

Brain dead indeed!

"Tom," I repeated. "Move your eyes up and down."

He did.

"Move them up and down twice if you understand me."

He did.

Once.

Twice.

"Side-to-side."

He did.

"Up and down means 'yes' and side-to-side means 'no.' Do you understand?"

Up and down.

He understood.

So did Frances. She was smiling, radiantly. She no longer looked out of style, or out of place. Woody Allen had been replaced by Alfred Hitchcock.

It did not take me long to piece it all together. Tom had been knocked out in the accident and had been unconscious when the police had found him. His heart had been beating.

An ambulance arrived. He wasn't breathing. The medics had put a tube down his throat.

Now he had recovered consciousness. But why had he stopped breathing?

The answer horrified me.

"Lift your right arm." I told him.

He couldn't.

Nor his left arm.

Nor either leg.

Tom Benton had a broken neck. That was why he couldn't breathe. He could not move any muscles below his neck.

And he couldn't talk because he had a breathing tube shoved down his throat.

The treatment for an acute neck injury is immediate immobilization. Every paramedic knows that. So does anyone who has ever taken any course in emergency health care. Any Boy Scout. But Tom's neck had not been immobilized.

Just the opposite.

I pictured him strapped into a Cessna as the air being pumped into him by the ambu flopped his head back and forth. Whatever chance he had had of recovering from his neck injury had undoubtedly been destroyed.

When had he regained consciousness?

Was he conscious in the plane?

Up and down.

In the ambulance?

Up and down.

When they put in the tube?

Side to side.

No. Sometime after the intubation. "Before they put you in the ambulance?"

Up and down.

"Did you see what the medics were saying?"

Up and down.

He began to cry.

"No one will take your heart," I said.

The crying continued.

The EEG tech began to detach the electrodes.

The chief of cardiac surgery walked over to us. "When can we have him?"

"Never," I said.

"Klawans, don't be obstructive," he said. "Just give us the damn heart."

"Go to hell." I explained.

The image of Tom Benton's head bouncing back and forth in a Cessna was still in my brain. A Cessna they had sent to pick him up.

Tom Benton was admitted to the neurosurgery service. They operated on him to immobilize his neck. Tom never got any better. He made no recovery. His spinal cord had been destroyed beyond recovery. He stayed in the ICU on a ventilator.

I never forgot him, but I stopped seeing him on rounds. I had nothing to offer him. Then one day I was in the surgical ICU seeing another patient, and noticed that he was not there. I asked the chief nurse what had happened.

"He died," she said.

"How?"

She shrugged. It had happened late one night. She didn't really know the details.

Pneumonia, I assumed. Or overwhelming infection. Or a pulmonary embolus—a blood clot to the lungs from the veins deep in his paralyzed legs. That can happen to severe quadriplegics who never get any better.

But I called the neurosurgeon and asked him.

"He died."

"How?"

He said nothing.

"Pneumonia?"

"No."

"Sepsis?"

"No."

"A pulmonary embolus?"

"No."

Were we playing twenty questions? If we were, I'd run out of questions.

I stopped.

After a pause, he went on. "His ventilator stopped."

"Those things don't just stop."

"They do if somehow it becomes unplugged."

He hung up.

We never again talked about Tom Benton, and I can no longer remember which team of cardiovascular surgeons performed the first cardiac transplant in Chicago. But I still remember Tom Benton.

23

WHAT I READ IN THE NEWSPAPERS

I only know what I read in the newspapers.

Will Rogers

It is not what a lawyer tells me I may do, but what humanity, reason and justice tell me I ought to do.

Edmund Burke

This also began with a phone call, to a resident in our pediatric ICU from an outside Emergency Room where they had a comatose baby. The baby had inhaled a balloon. Was there room in our pediatric ICU for another child?

There was, and the child became our patient. Unfortunately, the baby never woke up. He never regained consciousness. He remained in a coma, a permanent coma, but he was not brain dead. There were occasional squiggles on the EEG. Some meaningless movements of the eyes. Not much more. And it went on and on.

For days, for weeks, for months.

Coma vigil—a chronic vegetative state, the father was told. His son had become a vegetable. The vegetative functions of the body went on. The heart, the GI tract, the kidneys, the endocrine glands, even the lungs. Not the muscles that moved the air in and out. But as the ventilator moved the air, the lungs respired it. A chronic vegetative state.

The family could not take much more of that. Their son had suffered enough.

"Turn off the machines," the father pleaded.

The doctor said he couldn't do that.

Why not?

Because in doing so, he would be killing the little boy. And he could not do that. He had talked to the hospital's lawyers. They had told him that Illinois law only permits hospitals to withdraw life-support mechanisms from patients who have no brain activity, but that there was no precedent for what to do for patients who have minimal brain activity even if they have virtually no chance of regaining consciousness. The doctor felt he had no choice. He couldn't turn off the respirator. He had no right to do that.

The father went to see the hospital's lawyer. The lawyer told him that in order to protect the staff from potential criminal charges, the parents would have to go to court and have a judge issue a court order for removal of the respirator.

The father was not one for such legal niceties. He had no money. He was out of work. Where could he find a lawyer? Lawyers required money. Up front.

So one day he walked into his son's room in the pediatric ICU, pulled out a .357-caliber Magnum revolver, detached the respirator and cradled his fifteen-month old son in his arms until his son was dead. Then he gave up the body and the gun.

And he was arrested.

For murder.

Two weeks later, he was a free man. The grand jury refused to indict him for murder. Instead, he pleaded guilty to a misdemeanor—the unlawful use of a weapon. He was given a suspended sentence of one year.

I followed the story, like most other Chicagoans, by reading the newspapers. I never tried to see the child's chart. I had no right to do that.

I was horrified.

For the second time, I was ashamed of my own institution. The first time had been the death of Tom Benton. No lawyers had been involved then. This time, it was a nondeath. And too many lawyers had been involved this time.

Why, I wondered, had the baby been transferred here? We did not have the only pediatric ICU in town. Loyola had a pediatric ICU and was closer to the original hospital.

Loyola, I learned by reading the newspapers, had been asked but had refused to take the infant. Why? They felt he was already dead.

Was he?

236

That was what the medical examiner thought. He too, was quoted in all the newspapers. The father had not killed the child. You cannot kill someone who is already dead. And the child had died before he had ever entered that ER.

The baby had inhaled the balloon and lost consciousness. The family called the paramedics. They waited for the paramedics to arrive. After three minutes the father picked up his lifeless son and ran to the nearest hospital. It was at least a seven-minute run.

That meant at least ten minutes of no oxygen.

The baby's brain was already dead.

Why had we accepted him?

And why had we not just let him die? It had been more than a dozen years since the landmark Quinlan case in which the New Jersey Supreme Court had unanimously ruled that a patient in an irreversibly comatose state had the right to be free of any "extraordinary" medical intervention. Since then, almost a hundred state and federal courts had issued similar rulings. It was difficult for me to believe that the legal status of withdrawing a respirator from someone in a vegetative state could be in doubt in anyone's mind. Had I killed William Jessup? Should I have put him on a respirator?

He could still be alive today.

A vegetable.

So could George Gershwin.

I am not a lawyer, but it is an issue I have been following because death had become a neurologic diagnosis.

Two doctors in California had been charged with murder for withdrawing life-sustaining treatment from a comatose patient. A California court dismissed the charges and ruled that the cessation of "heroic" life-support measures is not an affirmative act of killing but rather a "withdrawal or omission of further treatment."

That had not been the only case. The U.S. District Court of Rhode Island had made a very similar ruling when it authorized the removal of artificial nutrition and fluid from a forty-nine-year-old woman in a persistent vegetative condition. "The issues presented do not essentially involve death, but essentially relate to life and its circumstances . . . ."

How could our lawyers have not known that? How could a spokesman from our institution insist that to "disconnect life-support would have amounted to at least child abuse under Illinois law"? Had no one here ever read the federal Baby Doe regulations of 1984? I had. They are quite explicit. "Withholding treatment is not medical neglect when the infant is chronically and irreversibly comatose."

Doctors make decisions to end life-sustaining treatment, including the removal of ventilator support from irreversibly comatose patients, every day without recourse to courts or legal proceedings or lawyers. I hope it stays that way.

24

THE GROUNDING OF THE PAINTED BIRD

I decided to devote my life to telling the story because I felt that having survived I owe something to the dead . . . and anyone who does not remember betrays them again.

Elie Wiesel

"But there won't be any more novels, Dad," she said. "He's dead. That's what got me started rereading his stuff."

"Dead," I gasped. My daughter's pronouncement caught me completely off guard. Jerzy Kosinski was dead. It wasn't the fact of a single death that distressed me; I'm used to hearing about deaths, witnessing them, recording them, certifying them. Deaths are part of my life. I long ago learned that everyone dies. But he was one of the actual witnesses, one of those who had somehow survived the Holocaust and had been transformed into living witnesses, sort of modern day Harpies whose roles in life are to make the world remember what had happened, what had been allowed to happen. Harpies didn't die. They kept to their unpleasant task. How could witnesses be allowed to die?

True, the first witness had died before her testimony ever became public. Anne Frank. She would have been only sixty-one, had she not been exterminated at the age of sixteen. Sixty-one. The average age of the onset of Parkinson's disease.

"When?" I finally managed to ask my daughter.

"A week ago. Didn't you know?"

"No."

I'd been in Europe on a whirlwind trip and I had, as my daughter so bluntly put it, "missed it" while I was away.

I could still see the cover of his first novel flashing in front of me. *The Painted Bird.* It has been published in 1965. Kosinski was in his early thirties then. That would make him under sixty now. Younger than Anne Frank. Younger than the average Parkinson's patient. Only a few years older than I was. And an infinitely better writer, with so much more to say.

I'd read *The Painted Bird* the year it had been published. I was in the army then, working as a neurologist in a hospital just outside Washington. The book was autobiographical. It was the story of a young Jewish boy, a Polish Jew, less than ten years old. His parents sent him to the Polish countryside in order to escape the Nazis. And he did escape them, but he was confronted by threats and violence of a far different sort. The boy, called Gypsy, was abandoned and wandered through a nightmarish world in which he was beaten, starved, brutalized, and tortured. Not by the Nazis, but by that world, a world of vicious, sadistic, and ignorant peasants.

And why?

Because he was there, and was not one of them.

Scene after scene conjured itself up in my mind. As fresh as if I had just put the book down. Other images also come back to me. Interviews with Kosinski. Reviews. Taunts.

"How had such things happened?" the world of nonvictims had asked in disbelief.

"Every incident is true," the witness had testified.

Right down to the garish bird painted on the wooden ceiling. A bird of prey that could swoop down and snatch away a life. Or that could soar above the rooftops away from the cruelties of mere humans. Ah, to be such a painted bird, to swoop, to soar.

And now Jerzy Kosinski was dead. He could no longer be a witness. His testimony was completed.

His other books were not about the Holocaust per se. Yet they were all the product of that experience, so how could they not reflect it?

Kosinski always remained a displaced person trying to survive in an unknown and hostile world not of his own; a true stranger in a strange land. People and critics call him paranoid. Just like many of his main characters. Not just Gypsy. But was he really paranoid?

Behaviorally, yes. Kosinski did not trust the world in which he found himself. He created false identities. He wore disguises. He had hiding places wherever he went. The world was not to be trusted.

But was that paranoia? True paranoia? Clinically, paranoia can only be diagnosed if the threat is not real or if the response is not realistic.

What, I ask, are the limits to the realistic responses to the Holocaust? Are there any?

His second book, *Steps*, was also derived from a life of violence in Poland. Polish violence toward someone who dared to be different. It won the National Book Award. Nothing else he wrote achieved that same level of critical reception.

"A first-class second-rate novelist" Kosinski had more than once called himself.

Yet he had always been a first-class witness. Right up there with Elie Wiesel, Anne Frank, André Schwartzbart.

And now he was dead.

"How?" I asked. How had the witness died?

"They found him in his bathtub."

A heart attack, I assumed. What ignominy. To survive the Holocaust to die in a bathtub. Why not? What could have been more normal? More peaceful. Too soon, but prosaic enough. No gas chamber. No oven. No ditch.

The survivor was gone. After surviving so much both physically and emotionally. He had even survived revisionism. He had been attacked viciously for being a witness. He had slandered Poland. There had even been a front page article in the *Village Voice* saying that he had not written *The Painted Bird*. If he hadn't, who the hell had? According to the revisionists *The Painted Bird* had been written by editors he had hired. Kosinski and the CIA. It was a lie so big that no sane man could possibly believe it. If such editors existed, I'd sure like to have them. So would untold thousands of other writers. And what else had they written? *The Last of the Just*? In French. *The Diary of a Young Girl*? In Dutch. Such talent. Such multilingual brilliance. How could any responsible editor publish such nonsense? Had the *Village Voice* ever apologized, ever retracted? I don't know. I simply give up reading it. Discrediting witnesses is the same as perpetrating the Holocaust. You have to stand up and be counted. For or against. There is no middle ground. You either attack the lie or become a part of it.

"Dad," she said. "He had one of your diseases."

"One of my diseases?" A neurologic disease. "Which one?"

"I'm not a neurologist," she protested, then added "the baseball one."

"Baseball . . . . You mean Lou Gehrig's disease."

"That's what I said. I think that's what the paper said."

ALS. Amyotrophic lateral sclerosis. A death sentence as sure as a train ride to Auschwitz. More certain. There were no survivors.

"It's a good thing he had a heart attack," I said.

"He didn't have a heart attack," she informed me.

"No heart attack?"

"No. Didn't you know? He killed himself. He tied a plastic bag over his head and—"

I only half heard the rest of what she said.

Society had gotten back at Jerzy Kosinski. What a way to die. He had ALS. That left him with two choices. A slow death or interruption of that process. The survivor had chosen the latter. To die as he wanted to die.

But why in a bathtub with a plastic bag over his head? Why had not his physician given him some sleeping pills? A simple OD had to be better than that. Why didn't physicians understand that? Why didn't our society?

"Too bad he wasn't your patient."

"What?"

"Grammie."

She was right. My mother and I had reached an agreement. She was eighty-seven. She had severe heart disease and could hardly leave her apartment. Her mind was intact, but her body was failing her. She never wanted to become dependent.

I understood that.

"I will never go into the hospital again," she said.

"But you will do everything else your doctor says, whatever he tells you to do."

"Yes," she promised. "And you will not let them put me into a hospital. I can die at home much more easily. And as myself. Not just some old lady being forced to live a life not worth living."

"Yes," I agreed.

"And I need a prescription for Seconal. I have trouble sleeping."

I gave her the prescription.

After she died, at home, of an acute myocardial infarction, we found two things in her apartment—the unused bottle of Seconal and half a dozen well-hidden boxes of hand-dipped chocolates which she had ordered and had delivered to her apartment. Not exactly what the doctor had ordered, but part of being independent and leading her own life.

Yes, I would have given Kosinski a prescription for sleeping pills. No witness deserves to have to die as he did.

Nor anyone else.

Life, Death, and in Between

Anne Frank, had she lived and remained in Amsterdam, could never have suffered the same fate as Jerzy Kosinski. True, she was attacked by revisionists. And she certainly could have developed ALS. Such neurologic problems may in fact be much more common in survivors who had lived through such untold deprivations. But in the Netherlands, physician-assisted suicide is legal, as is euthanasia of patients with terminal diseases. And the Netherlands is an entire country of survivors.

25

MEETING DOCTOR DEATH

God will forgive me . . . . That's His business.

Heinrich Heine

*The tears of the world are in constant quantity. For each one who begins
to weep, somewhere else another stops.*

Samuel Beckett
The Second Half

Geoff's a plaintiff's lawyer who specializes in medical malpractice. I've known him for over a decade, since I'd been the key expert
in his first major medical malpractice case. When that case came to
trial he won a million-dollar verdict, the first in his career, and we've
been on friendly terms ever since.

One day he called me. "I'm Kevorkian's lawyer," he said.

I didn't have to ask who Kevorkian was; his name had been all
over the TV news and newspapers for months. "Dr. Death," I replied.

"None other."

"Why you?" I inquired, not so innocently. The fact that they
were both from the Detroit area was not reason enough. Kevorkian
had been tried for murder. He'd needed a criminal attorney, not a civil
attorney, and Geoff, as far as I knew, limited his practice to civil cases.
Or had. I also knew that Geoff was a bit of a showman. And, of course,
Kevorkian was obviously not someone who wanted to avoid publicity. I'd seen him on TV more than once. I'd read the interviews he'd
given. He relished the publicity. Publicity was what he wanted.
Publicity for his cause. For the rights of patients to die when and
where and how they choose. And with the help of their own physicians. Or at least a physician of their own choice. When. Where. Why.
How. And with whose help. If the law didn't accept that, that was the
law's problem, not his. And he fought the medical establishments

whenever he could. Not just in their courts, behind their closed doors. He'd do it publicly. It wasn't just his own private crusade. It was a public one. And so Kevorkian's entire approach had been aimed at generating publicity, starting with his mercy machine. What else could explain that Rube Goldberg apparatus of his? Physicians have been quietly assisting patients to commit suicide since time immemorial. That was not enough for Jack Kevorkian. He had a bigger battle to fight. It was not his patient he needed to help, but all patients, of all doctors. Kevorkian, I reminded myself, was not a treating physician. He was a pathologist. He could not "help" patients as part of his ongoing care of them. In his usual line of work, they were already dead when they got to him. It's a different view of life and death.

"The Beaumont business," Geoff told me. "He remembered that and thought I'd be able to help him."

Geoffrey had once all but closed down Beaumont Hospital in Detroit because it refused to pay part of a malpractice judgment. Geoff Fieger had represented the plaintiff in a suit against Beaumont and had received a judgment of one and a quarter million dollars. The hospital, after all of its appeals had been exhausted, gave Fieger a check for part of the money, but refused to pay the last half a million dollars or so. It seems that they disagreed with the jury and felt the injuries weren't really worth one and a quarter million dollars. They obviously believed that Geoffrey would give in and negotiate with them and agree to accept a figure somewhat less that the original judgment. They had gravely misjudged their adversary. Fieger went into court and told the judge his story. The hospital, he complained, had no right not to pay the judgment. The judge agreed and so Fieger secured a writ of execution from the court, giving him the right to close down the hospital—an unprecedented decision. The hospital was like another business that was in default on a court-ordered judgment. So Fieger put together a group of deputy sheriffs and went to the hospital, accompanied, of course, by reporters and TV crews, intent on seizing the hospital's assets and shutting it down unless the hospital paid the money due his injured client. The hospital then gave him the check, right on the spot, TV cameras recording away.

Geoff was originally going to write "the book" about Kevorkian's case, but we decided that I should write it instead. The entire story. The building of the mercy machine. Meetings with the patient herself. Her side of the story. Her interviews with Kevorkian. His analysis. His response. The act itself. The physician-assisted suicide. And then the legal processes. Not just from the public court records but all of the behind-the-scenes machinations and maneuvers.

I would come up to Detroit for a weekend and meet with Geoff, Kevorkian, and the other principal participants to see if I could come up with an outline for a book about Kevorkian and Fieger. First, Geoff would send me all of the materials on Kevorkian and his twin cases, civil and criminal.

A few days later, the material arrived. I read it all, page after page, word for word. The details of the event itself were fairly easy to digest. At eight-thirty on the morning of June 4, 1990, Dr. Jack Kevorkian had driven his rust-eaten 1969 Volkswagen van into a rented parking space in a quiet park in Oakland County. Kevorkian had to be the only physician in America whose car was a beat-up '69 Volks. He obviously had not been in medicine for the money. At the same time, his two sisters, Flora and Margo, picked up his patient Janet Adkins at her hotel. Janet was not really his patient. They had no long-standing physician-patient relationship. She'd flown into Detroit from her home in Oregon just for this one meeting. She'd seen Kevorkian on TV; she knew that he offered her the help she needed. Janet had already written a brief note in which she spelled out her unswerving desire to end her own life. It was her choice and hers alone. She knew that she had Alzheimer's disease. A number of doctors had examined her and confirmed the diagnosis. Specialists. Neurologists. And she knew precisely what the future held out for her. That was not a future she could accept for herself or her family. She gave her handwritten note to Flora and with one last tearful farewell, said goodbye to her husband, Ron, and her best friend, Carol. They both had flown into Detroit with her. The morning was cold, damp, overcast. The threatening sky did not seem to promise good things to any of them.

While the three women were driving silently toward Grovelend Park, the site chosen for the physician-assisted suicide, Dr. Kevorkian, in the back of his van, nervously put his mercy machine through yet a few more test runs. Nothing could be allowed to go wrong. He had carried out hundreds of dry runs, practice runs, but never a real run-through, never a real performance with the machine pumping its solutions into an IV line that actually went into a patient. He engaged the switch and watched the chain as it turned the gears. Once. Twice. Three times. It seemed to be functioning perfectly. It had to. There could be no errors. No failures. It was all or nothing.

He decided to tighten the drive one more time, so he reached back in the cramped van for a pliers. His arm hit the container of thiopental, one of the three solutions that were the key to the success of his apparatus. It spilled. He tried to right it as quickly as he could; but over half of it was lost, spilled, gone. He had no extra bottles. He had thought that he had no need for spares. One vial was more than enough. But was half a bottle sufficient? How much thiopental did he need? How many milligrams per kilogram of body weight? What was her body weight? He'd never weighed her. He guessed. No more than sixty kilograms. Less. She was not a big woman.

He calculated. He had enough left. But could he be absolutely certain? He couldn't. They would have to drive back to his apartment in order to get another bottle.

It was at that point that Janet and the Kevorkian sisters arrived at the park. He told them what had happened. They were all upset by the mishap. Everyone's nerves were on edge. Everyone but Janet. She was the calmest of the four.

What should they do? They had no choice. They all drove back together to Kevorkian's apartment in Royal Oak to pick up a second vial of thiopental. His apartment, I later learned, was just a couple of sparsely furnished rooms over what was once a flourishing funeral home. It was close to noon when they finally got back to the park. The planned suicide, had it gone according to plan, should have long been over. The weather had not improved. It was still cold, overcast, and foreboding. The act should have been completed and they hadn't even started.

They parked. Janet remained in the car with Margo. Flora went into the van with her brother to assist him. She had never seen him so nervous.

Once again he tested his mercy machine. The machine is an electrically driven pump that pushes three fluids from their separate reservoirs through a single intravenous line into the patient. The first bottle contains thiopental, a rapidly acting barbiturate anesthesia which puts the patient into a deep coma, deep enough to stop all respiration; the second, succinylcholine, a curarelike agent to block all muscle activity and again paralyze all breathing; and the third, potassium chloride, which will stop the heart. Once the intravenous line is in place, the patient pushes the switch to turn the device on and initiate the entire process of anesthesia, paralysis, and death. In so doing, it is the patient who makes the final choices as to whether to perform the act of suicide and the exact moment at which to do the deed. Life and its termination remain under the control of the patient. A physician had designed the machine and shown the patient how to turn the switch on, but it was the patient's own acts that led to death. It was just what Kevorkian claims it to be, a suicide machine. Nothing more, nothing less. A lot less dangerous than a gun, or a gas oven, or a bottle of aspirin.

Once. Twice. He made yet a few more minor adjustments and then another test run. Followed by another adjustment. He had never been this compulsive and agitated before. He was finally satisfied. Ore was he too exhausted to make any more adjustments? His fingers were stiff. It was chilly inside the van; the heater hadn't worked in years. Besides, the motor was off. There was too much of a risk of carbon monoxide poisoning if he left the motor running. It was a bad joke. Carbon monoxide poisoning was a good way to go. He'd long considered setting up a mercy machine that produced carbon monoxide poisoning. It was so peaceful, and the corpse always looked so good; red lips, flushed cheeks. Some other time. He had to get back to work.

He loaded the three solutions: Thiopental, succinylcholine, potassium chloride. The fatal trio. Anesthesia, paralysis, cardiac standstill. An arrest of the heart in midbeat.

He was ready. The machine was ready. Janet Adkins had been ready for hours. It was almost two in the afternoon. He nodded to his sister, who then went to the car and told Janet that the machine was prepared.

Janet entered the van by herself, through the open sliding door, and lay fully clothed on the built-in bed Jack Kevorkian had covered with freshly laundered sheets. She rested her head on the clean pillow and got as comfortable as she could. The windows were covered with clean drapes. After asking Janet's permission, Dr. Kevorkian, for now he was her doctor, her physician, giving her the professional assistance she had requested, cut small holes in her hose at her ankles. He then attached electrodes for the electrocardiogram to her ankles and her wrists. Next he covered her body with a light blanket.

No one said a word. There was a nod here or there. A few gestures. Nothing more was needed. Janet had requested that Flora read her the brief note from her friend, Carol, and then read the Twenty-third Psalm. Flora read the note, then the psalm. Doctor Kevorkian then repeated his earlier instructions to Janet about how the device was to be activated and asked her to go through the motions.

His voice cracked. She smiled calmly, said "Thank you," and

demonstrated that she knew exactly what she had to do.

Next came the IV itself. Starting an IV was a routine medical procedure. All it involved was putting a needle into a vein. No big deal. First-year medical students learn the skill in a few minutes. Even the most clumsy students master it. He decided to start the IV on Janet's left arm, in front of the elbow. He took the needle in his hand. His hand shook violently. Janet Adkins smiled at him. He pushed the needle through her skin, then into the vein and right on through it. Her blood oozed out of the vein and spread in the soft tissues under her skin. He had failed on his first attempt.

He pulled the needle out and made a second try. It turned out no better than the first. A third. He again missed the vein.

He shifted to the right side. A fourth attempt. A fifth. Had any medical student ever been this clumsy? This inept? He had never been. He was finally in the vein. The IV was running.

The time was at hand.

Dr. Kevorkian looked at Janet. She knew. She was ready. She nodded ever so slightly. Dr. Kevorkian turned on the EKG machine in order to monitor her heartbeat, to document her cardiac standstill, her arrest in midsystole. The EKG began to record each and every one of her heartbeats.

Janet activated the mercy machine. The fluids began to flow through the tubing and then into her vein. First one, then the next, then the third. Thiopental. Succinylcholine. Potassium chloride. A few moments later, ten, perhaps fifteen seconds, her eyelids began to droop. "Thank you," she said, "Thank you."

"Have a nice trip," Dr. Kevorkian replied.

Her eyes closed for the last time. Then her breathing slowed, it became more and more shallow. Never labored, never gasping, just slower, more shallow. Then gone. Not even a whimper. Just peace.

Six minutes after she had closed her eyes for the last time the complexes being traced out by the EKG flattened into a straight line. Jack Kevorkian breathed a sigh of relief. The EKG showed the flat line of cardiac standstill. It was all over. Janet Adkins was dead. He could feel his body begin to relax. He took a deep breath, a sigh of relief and as he did he glanced once again at the flat line of black ink rolling out of the EKG machine, the flat line of cardiac arrest. But it wasn't flat. There was a bleep. That wasn't supposed to happen. Flat was supposed to stay flat. Dead is dead. One little bleep. One beat of the heart. The second, a third.

"My God!" he screamed. Something was wrong. Her heart was

beating. Something had gone wrong. What? How? She was not breathing. She was not struggling. She was . . . dead. She had to be.

He stared back at the EKG. The line was flat. As flat as flat could be.

The beats, a few last agonal discharges of the heart, had disappeared. They were gone and Janet Adkins was dead.

How often, he wondered, had people died with a "thank you" on their lips? Not very often, he was sure. Especially not in hospitals. I, too was certain of that.

That could have been the end of the story. But it wasn't. It was more like the beginning. Within days, Dr. Kevorkian was in court, first in a civil courtroom, facing a permanent injunction against advocating physician-assisted suicide, even against just discussing suicide with patients, and certainly against advising anyone on the use of the mercy machine, and of course a permanent bar on using the machine. Meanwhile, the sale of guns was still legal in Michigan. And Dr. Kevorkian also faced charges in a criminal courtroom. He was charged with first-degree murder. Yet Janet Adkins had committed suicide. She had not flown to Detroit with her husband and best friend because Jack Kevorkian was some evil Rasputin who had drawn her in to kill her.

The details of the court cases were more complicated than what had happened to Janet Adkins that afternoon. They were far more convoluted, more technical. They involved more than a simple machine and three solutions. And more than just one out of work pathologist. These I'd have to discuss further with Fieger and his co-counsel. But it looked like this was a story well worth telling. Two stories in fact. Jack Kevorkian's story, his battle for the rights of patients, and Fieger's battle for Kevorkian's rights.

Two separate battles, two crusades.

But what about the leading character? What was Kevorkian really like?

He'd written a book about those issues that had always interested him as an individual human being and as a pathologist, *Prescription Medicide*. Reading his own words made me realize that Kevorkian was a man who had always been obsessed with death. No single patient, tale of horror, or single tragedy, had gotten him involved in physician-assisted suicide. That did not really surprise me; after all, he had chosen to become a pathologist, not a bedside physician. He never watched his patients die. He held no hands. They were already dead before he met them. What little research he had done had centered around death—determining how long a body had been dead, using blood from cadavers in transfusions into living beings. Doctor Death. Over the years he'd become more and more angered by society's refusal to accept death and the suffering that that refusal caused. He'd spent most of his professional life attempting to change the ways, the means, and the meaning of death. His philosophy included much more than just physician-assisted suicide. Planned suicide was only a starting point. Another of the problems he cared about was the right of executed criminals to donate their organs for medical uses, which is now illegal. A criminal is electrocuted in order to pay a debt to society and that man or woman cannot donate his or her organs. Are we afraid that those kidneys will turn the recipient into a twentieth-century Frankenstein?

Kevorkian was right. No rational human being could disagree. Only fifty state legislatures and fifty governors.

He also advocates the right of such criminals to choose to undergo medical experimentation under general anesthesia, instead of traditional execution. This one was a bit too much for me to swallow, but still it was worth discussing. Then there was the possibility of using cadaver blood for transfusions. He'd even done some research. If possible and safe, an army in the field might have all the blood it would need. Grotesque perhaps. Immoral, unethical? Of course not. He was also in favor of the sale of organs for transplantation. That was another place where we disagreed, but he had some valid arguments which were well worth hearing and considering.

There was more than a grain of truth in much of what he wrote. But the whole was more than just the sum of its parts. Like all polemicists he used a lot of hyperbole and had a somewhat paranoid view of the world, which he saw as a hostile place in which he had long been fighting a heroic lonely crusade for truth and justice.

I became convinced that Jack was a true believer, a crusader without armor. He took on the medical establishment, the legal system, and many aspects of our society because he thought they were wrong. It was him against them, a fight to the end. He had more than just a touch of Don Quixote in him.

His life had not been an attempt to gain glory. Medicine had plenty of ways to obtain glory. Kevorkian had followed none of these pathways.

In rereading his book it became very clear that despite his attempts, Kevorkian was not a scholar. He used secondary sources and was often satisfied with rather superficial, perfunctory summaries of that data that fit into his view of the world. One of his big errors stood out like a sore thumb in the chapter in which he expounded his concept of experimentation on condemned criminals. He called the chapter "Nothing New Under the Sun" and in it he traced the long history of such experiments from Hellenistic Alexandria, well over two thousand years ago, up to the twentieth century. He then focused on the experimentation done on Armenians by the Turks and those done by the Nazis on Jews. Confusing such atrocities on victims of genocide with voluntary participation in experimentation by condemned criminals disturbed me. He then compounded that by stating that some of the results of the experiments carried out by Nazi physicians on helpless prisoners in concentration camps were of "considerable scientific value." His example of this was the infamous "research" on cold-water survival. The cold-water immersion project was conducted at the Dachau concentration camp between 1942 and 1943. It had ostensibly been done to establish the most effective treatment for victims of sudden lowering of body temperature due to immersion in very cold water. German interest in this problem had been stimulated by the shooting down of many German airmen into the cold waters of the North Sea. The subjects in these "experiments" were all men: Jews, Poles, Czechs, and some Russian prisoners of war. Their participation in the experiment was forced. The occasional "voluntary" participation was the product of promises of release from the camp or commutation of the death sentence once the experiments were over. Such promises were not kept, and there was no informed consent.

During the experiments, the subjects were put into a tank filled with ice-cold water. Some were anesthetized, but most were fully conscious. Many were naked, but others were clothed. Several different methods of rewarming the subjects were also tested. What happened to the subjects' body temperatures, their symptoms, and some selected biochemical and physiologic measurements were reportedly monitored. And autopsies were performed, of course.

Such experiments certainly transgressed both human decency and the Helsinki Convention for protection of human rights. As such, most editors of real medical journals will not even permit mention of the results in their journals. The Helsinki Convention forbids the use of such data. This infuriated Kevorkian. It was good research, it should be part of our usable database. That knowledge could save lives. He then took off on those editors: they had now created a new ethical "crisis" by rejecting all such references because of the unethical circumstances involved in the attainment of the data cited. "But in thus arbitrarily denying the validity of, and access to, legitimate and useful medical information, our esteemed editors are as guilty of moral infraction as were their counterparts in Nazi Germany who equally arbitrarily forbade their medical students from citing Jewish references in their doctoral dissertations."

I was stunned. First by his moral standard. Comparing the ethics of the likes of Josef Mengele with those of editors who refused to publish references to their data. Could he really believe that? The second reaction was less emotional, but more bothersome in its own way. The cold-water research was worthless. How could anyone be foolish enough to stick his neck out to defend it? The experimenters were not great scientists. Their work was not done under controlled conditions. Their population was not healthy to begin with. The so-called investigators were sadistic men whose judgment was colored by their own hatreds. More to the point, a recent article on the Dachau hypothermia experiments in the *New England Journal of Medicine* by Robert L. Berger had pinpointed all the reasons why the data were seriously flawed from a scientific viewpoint. The experiments had not been performed in any scientific manner. The data were riddled with inconsistencies as well as apparent falsification and, most likely, out-and-out fabrication. Many of the so-called conclusions were not supported by the actual observations. The flawed science was further compounded by evidence that the director of the project had throughout his career displayed a consistent pattern of dishonesty and deception that characterized both his professional and his personal life, a man who could not be trusted to recognize the truth, much less tell it. Berger had quite clearly stripped this so-called study of the last vestige of credibility. How could Kevorkian ignore this article?

Had Kevorkian studied the original experiments and the reports? I searched his bibliography for Berger's report. It was not there. How could he have missed it? The *New England Journal of Medicine* is not an obscure source. Had he read the 1946 report by Leo Alexander? Alexander had studied the experiments in detail and concluded that they were not dependable. I could not understand how Kevorkian had somehow jumped on the bandwagon of insisting that such atrocities could result in good.

The next weekend my wife and I drove to Detroit. In the afternoon, I talked with Geoff about the two cases and the legal issues. That night we all met for dinner—Geoff and his wife, my wife and I,

Jack Kevorkian and one of his sisters. Jack struck me as a bantam rooster. Thin, wiry, gray-haired, a Jacques Cousteau with somewhat heavier facial features. He also had an obvious warmth and empathy. This was not a man who could ever hurt another human being. But he was also volatile. The evening started off well enough. We talked baseball. He was an old Detroit Tiger fan. I'm a White Sox fan, but misspent my youth memorizing the baseball encyclopedia. We seemed to hit it off.

As dinner went on, we got into more serious discussion. Janet Adkins. He became more and more animated. Angry. Critics had been attacking his clinical judgment.

Why?

He had no proof that she was competent to decide for herself on her course of action. After all, she had Alzheimer's disease. Perhaps she was too demented?

"No proof," he spouted. "I talked to her for two days."

"Did you do a Mini Mental Status?"

"A what?"

Perhaps I shouldn't have been surprised. Everyone who works with patients with dementia does a Mini Mental Status on each patient as part of routine medical care. It's automatic. It is a series of questions that covers basic mental functions and is quantified, reliable, reproducible, and respected. And he hadn't done one. If he had and she'd scored well, then he couldn't be criticized. He'd never heard of it.

Why was I surprised? He was a pathologist. Pathologists don't practice medicine. He hadn't even worked as a pathologist for almost a decade.

I explained the Mini Mental Status to him. He seemed interested. I'd send him the form. But he should have known about it. Anyone dealing with Alzheimer's disease should. Didn't he keep up with the literature? Then I remembered. Dachau. Berger. I shifted the conversation to human experimentation. Voluntary experimentation on condemned criminals.

Involuntary.

World War II.

The Holocaust.

Dachau.

And there he was attacking all those stupid editors who were killing people by suppressing valuable information.

What valuable information?

The freezing experiments.
Had he read them?
No.
Had he read Alexander's report?
Yes.
"Berger's?"
He'd never heard of him. He'd lauded the data based on secondary sources, from rumor. He'd ignored Alexander and not even bothered to read the most recent articles. He was certainly not a scholar. But neither was Don Quixote.

I should have stopped there. I couldn't. There is more than a touch of Don Quixote in me, too.

I attacked.

He counterattacked.

The evening ended not with a peace treaty, but merely a cease-fire. As Geoffrey waited for his car I told him that Kevorkian had better edit that material out of his book. If not, reviewers could kill him. Our cause was too important.

"But he only does what he really believes."

"I know," I replied. "That's why I want to write the book."

I had met Doctor Death. And he was part hero and part non-hero. Is any hero ever more than that?

I was ready to start the book.

Two weeks later, I got a call from Geoff. Kevorkian had asked him to call me.

Why?

Two reasons. First, could I send him a Mini Mental Status form? I could. What was the second?

Kevorkian wanted me to know that he had deleted all reference to the freezing experiments from his book.

"So I convinced him."

"Not really."

"What do you mean."

"He'd already changed it. You had the first set of proofs. That was only an argument he'd tried out and then rejected on his own. It appealed to his anti-establishment bias. But he'd changed it in the next draft."

"Then why did we have that argument?"

"He loves a good fight."

Kevorkian's story has not ended. A judge threw out the murder charge. There had been no murder. It had been a suicide, a physician-assisted suicide. Janet Adkins had wanted to commit suicide and she'd succeeded. Kervorkian had helped her but so what? There's no law against that in Michigan.

Jack had won that round. But not just for himself. For a lot of other people. Maybe. Janet Adkins had decided that she wanted to die. She had a terminal illness, and in its inexorable progress she chose suicide. The prosecution tried to call it murder and failed. The rights of patients with terminal diseases to control their own lives and their own deaths had come out of the closet and onto TV screens, just where Jack Kervorkian wanted it to be. The first round was over, but not the fight.

Round two began on October 23, 1991, a cold Fall morning, in an isolated cabin in a state park outside Detroit. This time Jack assisted in a double suicide. One woman had severe multiple sclerosis. MS is a potentially terminal illness, but the course is very erratic and difficult to predict with any accuracy. Unlike Alzheimer's disease, it's not inexorably progressive.

Who knows how long she had to live? She didn't. Her neurologists didn't. Kevorkian didn't. But she didn't want to go on. She was completely incapacitated. She wanted to kill herself. And to Kevorkian she too had the right to die, when, where, and how she wanted to—a bigger challenge to societal norms that Janet Adkins.

And what about the other woman? She had severe pain that had required ten surgical procedures, but no terminal illness. Just a long lifetime of pain that no one could make go away. Pain with a normal life expectancy. She too turned to Jack and he didn't turn away.

Round two. Two women who wanted to commit suicide and on videotape told the world what they wanted to do and why and when and how. Jack was the only one who would help them.

And he did. With lots of witnesses.

And the state called it murder. A grand jury indicted him for murder.

Once again Geoff defended him. In court, on "20/20," on "Phil Donahue." Two crusaders doing what they do best and doing it publicly as they could.

26

THE ELEVENTH
COMMANDMENT

If I am not for myself, who is for me? And being for my own self, what am I? And if not now, when?

Hillel the Elder
70 B.C.E.—10 C.E.

As I walked from my office to the hospital, I realized that this had to be the first time I had made rounds as a attending physician on the consultation service in over a year. Longer than that, in fact. It was actually closer to two years since I had last been responsible for seeing all of the neurologic consultations in the hospital. That long a lapse did not bother me. I was certain that neurology hadn't changed very much, nor had the way one teaches or practices medicine. There would be some changes: New antibiotics, new protocols for the treatment of some cancer or other, new neurologic manifestations of AIDS. But overall, little would have changed. Patients would still be suffering from the same diseases and those diseases would still be diagnosed in the same way. A seizure would still be a seizure, a stroke would still be a stroke.

The residents had three patients for me to see. The first was a woman in her forties with widespread cancer of the breast. Her cancer had not responded to any of the usual forms of treatment. She wanted the doctors to try everything and anything. They did. According to the resident, she'd been put onto a "salvage" protocol.

"What is that?" I inquired, trying not to seem too out of date.

"Well," she began, "The routine protocols had all failed. The usual doses of anticancer drugs hadn't touched her. In this protocol, the patient is given toxic doses of several of those drugs, large enough to be fatal. The hope is that that amount of medicine will kill the cancer cells and that we can then save her by use of antibiotics, bone marrow transplants . . . whatever has to be done."

I nodded slowly.

"That's why it's called *salvage*," she continued. "We try to salvage her out of the destruction we caused."

I nodded again, very half-heartedly, already feeling either out of date or out of step. Or both.

The resident went on to outline the rest of the patient's story. It was a relentless saga of the known complications of excessive chemotherapy. A series of infections. Liver failure. Anemia. Spontaneous bleeding.

And then the patient had lapsed into coma.

"Why?" As I asked the question, I had imagined my own list of diagnostic possibilities. The most probably causes were both related to her chemotherapy. One would be an infection such as meningitis caused by the damage her medications had done to her ability to ward off infections. The other would be a massive hemorrhage into the brain, a hemorrhage made possible by the same poisons that had destroyed her ability to produce those substances which keep normal people from bleeding spontaneously.

"She bled into her brain."

I knew the entire scenario. Chemotherapy. Suppression of her bone marrow. Lack of normal clotting factors. Spontaneous bleeding.

Cerebral hemorrhage.

Coma.

Death.

An iatrogenic death. There was not much to do once this had occurred. This was one of the complications with a very low salvage rate.

They showed me the CAT scan.

I'd been too optimistic. She had had two massive hemorrhages, not just one, with a marked degree of brain damage. The salvage rate would be zero, at best. If she survived, she'd have severe brain damage.

But her doctors were still treating her as aggressively as possible. The salvage effect, once started, had a momentum of its own.

More problems developed.

She had no white blood cells. She developed a series of infections. She was given massive doses of antibiotics and when that failed, experimental antibiotics—and God knows what else. By that time, both my tolerance for such idiocy and my attention span had been exceeded.

Her physicians had asked someone from neurology to see if she should be put on anticonvulsant medications to prevent the possibility that her hemorrhage could lead to a seizure.

"Why are we doing all of this?" I exploded.

"Because she asked us to. She told us to," the resident explained. "She told us to do everything possible."

"How often do we do such things?" I went on. "Salvage protocols?"

"A couple a month."

"I've never seen one. For how long?"

"About a year."

That explained why I'd never seen such a patient. But we'd done a couple of dozen. "Have any of them been cured?"

The resident had never seen one.

I went to the ICU and examined the patient. She was in a coma. Other than responding to pain, moving her eyes from time to time and triggering her ventilator every once in a while, her brain could do nothing. She'd been like that for over a week. She'd never get any better. As far as I was concerned, she didn't need anticonvulsant medication. She needed to be allowed to die.

The consultation request asked a simple question.

"Will this patient profit by being on anticonvulsants?"

I gave a simple response. My entire note consisted of one word. "No."

The second patient I had been asked to see was a fifty-seven-year-old man. He'd been in the hospital for almost five months. He was a VIP. Over the last decade he'd given the hospital over a million dollars. He had chronic liver failure and a tumor of the liver. Five months ago, he'd come in for a liver transplant. He'd gotten that transplant and quickly rejected it.

Within a few days of that rejection, another liver had been located, and the patient had once again undergone the same surgical procedure. New liver for old. Out with the bad liver, in with the new one. Transplant number two.

He'd also rejected that liver, just about as quickly as he'd rejected the first one.

But medical progress didn't stop there. After all, these had not been the only two livers in the world.

I knew exactly what had happened next. Transplant number three.

This was the one he was now rejecting. In addition, his liver tumor was now spreading. It now involved more than just the area of the abdominal wall which housed each of his succession of ill-fated livers. Tumors were now invading his skin, his lungs, his stomach.

"God," I mused aloud, "may be telling us something."

The resident ignored my comment. He apparently had little interest in God's warnings.

The resident continued his recitation, as irreverent as ever. It was obvious that the resident was not the only one who was unwilling to give any credence to the events of the past. The patient shared his feeling. As did the rest of the medical staff. There had to be more that could be done. The fact that this man's body had destroyed four healthy livers didn't stop them. And that he had a metastatic cancer for which we had no cure seemed to mean nothing.

I shuddered at the prospect of yet another salvage protocol. Why not? The patient wanted no stone left unturned. Even his own gravestone. He couldn't be given another liver. Not while his liver cancer was spreading like wild fire. A transplant wouldn't stop that.

"So what did they do?" I asked, more than half afraid of the answer.

"We gave him Tylenol in large amounts, intravenously. We gave him a dose far greater than is required to kill his liver," the resident informed me.

"Why?" I inquired, not so innocently. After all, I understood that Tylenol was a liver toxin. In large doses, it attacks the liver cells. The damage it causes is irreversible.

"We figured that the Tylenol would kill off the liver and then the transplant reaction would end and we could give him another liver. That one might even survive if there's a hiatus between the end of the rejection process for number three and the next transplant."

That *might* left one problem still unsolved.

"If," he added, "it kills off the tumor, too."

That sounded like a very big if to me. "The cancer cells were liver cells or at least had started life as liver cells. Tylenol might kill them, but would it?" I asked. According to the resident, no one knew if it would.

Had this been tried before?

No.

Why now?

"The patient wants us to do everything."

Did anyone really believe it would work?

"It might," someone said.

The third patient had AIDS. He too, had wanted no stone unturned and had told that to his physician in no uncertain terms. He wanted no treatment to go untried. Then the patient had lapsed into a coma.

When had that happened, I inquired.

Six weeks earlier.

And God only knew how many protocols and complications had transpired in those six weeks. After three weeks, which took fifteen minutes for the resident to summarize, I lost count.

I was fairly certain that I could not help this man.

As far as I was concerned, none of us could help him. Not in the way he had once wanted; not in the way they were trying.

It was time to quit. He'd been a coma for six weeks. For most of that time, it must have been abundantly clear to everyone, from the medical students on up, that the game was over. Victory had eluded them, and an unending tie was helping no one. Why had it gone on this long? Why was it still going on? The agonal phase of life should be kept as short as possible. Prolonging life should not consist of prolonging the final agony. There was no future in that. No worthwhile purpose was served. No one was helped. Not the patient. And not the next patient. What had medicine come to?

"Why are we doing this?" I shouted out, only then realizing that I had not just been cogitating to myself. I have been berating them all.

And they all thought I was out of date, I was wrong.

Why?

It was what the patient wanted. He had made a specific request and that request to them had the force of law. It was as if it had become the Eleventh Commandment. They had no choice in the matter.

"The patient has a right!" the resident argued.

"True. He has the absolute right to accept or reject anything his doctor suggests. And that may have the force of a commandment. But I have the same rights. The patient cannot tell me to do things I don't believe in. He can't tell me how to practice medicine. That's both my right and my obligation."

"What do you do if he says, 'Do everything' and you think nothing will help?"

"If there is nothing more to do that in my best judgment is

worthwhile doing, I do nothing."

"But the patient wants something done."

"He can find a different sucker. Not me. I can't force my patient to do what I think is proper. And he can't force me to do what I think is improper. I practice medicine the way I feel it should be practiced, not the way some frightened, dying, desperate patient demands. That's craziness."

The argument went on.

All in all, it was the least satisfying set of teaching rounds I'd ever given. No one had learned anything. No patient had been helped.

The next day we met for rounds again. It felt more like the beginning of round two of a heavyweight grudge match. Ali versus Frazier or Louis versus Schmelling. But it was more than two individual heavyweights at stake. It was a concept of life, of right and wrong. Of morality. Of the ethics of medicine.

We started rounds by reviewing what had happened to the three patients we'd seen during round one. There had been no changes, either in the patients or in everyone's attitudes.

We had two new consults to see; one had Parkinson's disease and one a stroke. There were no controversies. I wanted to ask them about the history of medical ethics. About the Oath of Hippocrates which they had all taken. According to that oath, their first obligation was to do no harm. Even if it was an oath to Apollo, the thesis was correct.

Round three took place the next morning.

Same contestants. Same atmosphere. I started by telling them a story about a patient I had helped treat. It had taken place during my internship.

Ten days before he died, all of us who were taking care of Peter Zale knew that there was nothing whatsoever that we could do to prevent his death. He was thirty-seven years old and had been in good health until just four weeks previously, and now we were going to watch him die. His own physician knew that; so did all the consultants and residents. Even I recognized the fact. No one had made an announcement. Or put a notice on his chart. Nothing so formal. Our revelation had come in the guise of a simple report from the hospital's infectious disease laboratory. Peter Zale's final pronouncement came on a single slip of paper with a list of seven Rs.

Peter Zale was a steelworker from the South Side of Chicago.

Like Tony Zale, the ex-middleweight boxing champion. His father, like Tony's, had also worked in the steel mills. And like the other Zale family, they had come to the United States from Poland and changed their name. The two families weren't related. They originally had different names. I don't recall what those names were and doubt if I ever knew how to pronounce them correctly, much less spell them.

Mr. Zale had told me that story on the evening of his admission. He was proud of his heritage. Proud of Tony Zale. Proud to be a Polish-American. Proud to be a steelworker. It was 1962 and he lived and worked in Chicago, the city with the second largest Polish population in the entire world—second only to Warsaw, more than Krakow. Had I known that?

"No," I readily admitted, anxious to get on to those facts that had brought Mr. Zale, of the longer and harder-to-pronounce name, into the hospital. He was only one of the six new admissions I had to see and examine that evening.

"What," I asked, "brought you to the hospital?"

Peter Zale had felt fine, perfect in fact, until about four weeks before. Then one day at work, he just didn't feel right. He felt weak and tired. When he finished his shift, he was exhausted. He was supposed to go bowling that night with some pals, but he was just too tired to go. A good night's sleep would fix him up. It always did. He'd been working too hard: sixty hours a week.

He went to bed at seven and his wife got him up at seven in the morning. Twelve hours of uninterrupted sleep. He felt better, not "in the pink," but better. He went to work and came home after his eight-hour shift exhausted. No Blackhawk hockey game for him. His friends were amazed. He hadn't missed a hockey game in a decade, and the Hawks were in the playoffs. That was like missing a Zale title fight.

"Not really," he'd told them. "To miss that I'd have to be six feet under," he'd laughed.

Each day his tiredness got worse. That weekend all he did was hang around the house. On Sunday night, his wife took his temperature. It was 100.4.

Monday he was no better.

Nor Tuesday.

And each evening, he had a slight fever.

His appetite wasn't what it had been. He'd lost four or five pounds.

Wednesday he stayed home from work and just lounged in bed all day. He had soup for dinner. That tasted good. But by 7:00 P.M., he was far too tired to watch the Hawks game on TV.

Thursday he again skipped work, but his wife took him to the doctor.

His blood pressure was fine.

So was his heart.

And his belly.

Still Peter had had a fever every night for almost a week.

"A virus," the doctor pronounced as he gave him a shot of penicillin and a prescription for more.

Peter got no better.

The next Monday, he went back to see the doctor. He still had the same symptoms.

Extreme fatigue.

Loss of appetite.

Low fever.

"A persistent virus," the doctor said, and increased the dose of penicillin, giving him two shots this time.

By Friday Peter was worse. He now got short of breath whenever he did anything, even just the short walk out to the mailbox at the corner. And he couldn't take the garbage out into the alley. The can was too heavy to lift. But he'd been doing that since he was ten years old.

He went to a new doctor. The doctor examined him, listened to his chest, looked into his throat, nodded sagely and said something about a new type of virus from Hong Kong.

Peter had never been to Hong Kong. He never left the South Side, except to go to Wrigley Field to root for the Chicago Bears.

According to this doctor, Peter needed a different antibiotic. The doctor put him on Terramycin, one of the newest of the miracle drugs, newer than penicillin. The doctor was certain that this would help. Peter hoped he was right, but what did he know about foreign viruses?

The Terramycin didn't help. Nor did the Erythromycin that was added a few days later. Peter's fatigue continued. So did his fever, loss of appetite, weight loss, shortness of breath. To these were added a couple of other problems; sweating and swelling of the feet. Obviously this new doctor didn't know much more about treating un-American viruses than he did. He needed another doctor, one who knew more about such viruses. His neighbor recommended a Dr. Phillips who had almost saved his aunt's life. Dr. Phillips wasn't just another neighborhood GP. He had an office downtown and he didn't send his patients to one of the small neighborhood hospitals. He admitted his patients to Presbyterian–St. Luke's Hospital.

That, Peter realized, was almost as far away as Wrigley Field. But what choice did he have?

That's how Peter Zale became my patient. He saw Dr. Norman Phillips in his office on Michigan Avenue. Phillips took his history, examined him, made a tentative diagnosis, told Peter that he did not have a virus. He had a serious bacterial infection involving his heart and needed to be in the hospital. That evening Peter was admitted to our hospital, to my service, and became my patient. After I concluded taking his history and examining and writing up my notes, I called Dr. Phillips to discuss the case. "Well, Professor," he began. Phillips called all interns Professor until they proved to him that they were good enough to be called Doctor. "What do you think of our patient?"

"He's a very sick man," I began tentatively.

"I don't admit well people, only sick patients, Professor."

That much I knew.

"Can you tell me in what particular way he's sick?"

I thought I could. Mr. Zale had a four-week history of an infection with fatigue, fevers, weight loss, and other such nonspecific complaints and a two week history of more specific complaints.

"Such as?"

"Shortness of breath and swelling of the feet."

"So how to you put that all together, Professor?"

"SBE," I proposed. SBE stands for subacute bacterial endocarditis, a bacterial infection in which the bacteria grow on one of the valves of the heart. Once there, the bacteria destroy the valve, causing a heart murmur and then heart failure with shortness of breath and build-up of fluid in the legs and lungs.

"Tell me, Doctor, how do we prove that?"

"He should have a new heart murmur."

"Does he?"

"I heard it."

"Did he ever have it before?"

"No other doctors ever told him about it."

"How loud is it?"

"If I heard it, it's probably too loud for anyone to miss," I told him.

"Then it must be new. So we know what he has. But what do we do, Doctor?"

267

"We have to find out exactly what kind of bacteria are growing on his heart and then which antibiotic will work to kill those bacteria."

"How do we do that?"

"Blood cultures," I replied. That meant drawing samples of blood under sterile conditions and sending them to the infectious disease laboratory.

"How many?"

"Six, and then I'd start him on IV penicillin and chloromycetin while the lab is getting us the answer."

Phillips agreed. I would draw the blood cultures over the evening and night.

Peter Zale needed the good fortune to have bacteria that would respond to one of our antibiotics. By six in the morning, I had sent off all six blood cultures, started the IV, and begun him on two of the most powerful antibiotics we had, penicillin and chloromycetin, fondly known as Pen and Chloro.

The first of the culture results came back two days later. Peter Zale's luck had not been good. The bacteria eating up the valve of his heart and causing his heart failure were called pseudomonas. That was a rare cause of SBE, and a very bad one. Pseudomona was a very hardy bacterium. Most antibiotics never phased it. It would take another twenty-four hours to see if his luck had been all bad.

That was how long it would take the lab to test his pseudomonas against all available antibiotics.

We waited and hoped, to no avail.

The slip came back the next day. It consisted of two columns. The first listed the antibiotics in alphabetical order and the second consisted of a single letter. Either S for sensitive, meaning the antibiotic would work, because the bacteria were sensitive to it, or R for resistant.

Peter Zale had a column of Rs. His pseudomona was not sensitive to penicillin or chloromycetin, the two drugs which we were using to treat him. It wasn't even sensitive to our most potent and dangerous antibiotic, amphotericin B, fondly called ampho-terrible by all the interns who had to monitor its effects on patients' kidneys and livers.

All Rs.

That left us no alternatives. There was nothing to do. Nothing would work. The pseudomonas would continue to eat away his valve and his heart would finally give out.

There had to be something to do.

But what?

We all felt like professors.

That afternoon, Dr. Robert M. Kark, one of our senior attending physicians, spend an hour making teaching rounds with the residents, interns, and medical students on our ward. He discussed half a dozen of our more challenging patients with us. Peter Zale was one of them.

I asked Dr. Kark if he could think of anything else we could do for Mr. Zale.

Offhand, he couldn't.

"Anything at all," I pleaded. "He is being overwhelmed by bacteria we can't treat."

Dr. Kark started talking about the history of SBE. The first description of the disorder, the first successful treatment, the miracle of penicillin.

None of this was helping Peter Zale.

Then he branched out to talk about the history of infectious diseases, of plagues. And then he stopped in midsentence. "There is one thing we could try. Pseudomona is a peculiar bacteria. It grows where there are no other bacteria, but only there. That means that even if we can't kill it, other bacteria can. So all we have to do is give your patient some other bacteria, one that is sensitive to penicillin, have that bacteria take hold on his heart valve, overgrow and kill off the pseudomonas and then we can treat that bacteria with penicillin."

Everyone was stunned. No one had ever heard of such an approach.

Dr. Kark admitted that it was unorthodox.

Unorthodox! It was absolutely radical in most of the residents' minds.

Dr. Kark didn't think it was that radical. It was one of the classical approaches to plagues.

I stopped telling my story and waited for a comment. It didn't take very long.

"You were no better than we are. No different. That's as crazy as anything we're doing."

"No," I replied, "there were two differences."

"What two differences?"

"We thought about this radical treatment because we were considering our options, not because the patient told us we had to do everything possible."

He was not impressed. "And what was the other difference?"

"We never did it. We just thought about it."

Round three was over.

Round four was very brief. It took place several days later. All three patients had died; the woman who had not been salvaged, the rich donor who had rejected three livers, and the man with AIDS.

I made no comment. My criticism filled the room nonetheless.

"And what happened to your patient?" the resident demanded. "To Mr. Zale?"

"He died."

"So what's the difference?"

"I never contributed to that death. He didn't bleed into his head because I killed off his bone marrow with my treatment and caused him to bleed. He didn't have total death of his partially rejected liver because I gave him a poison that I knew would kill his liver and hoped would kill his cancer."

I stopped. These were not the real issues.

"Mr. Zale died. But I did not hasten that death. And I did not uselessly prolong his agony. Believe it or not, all patients die. So do all doctors. It is one fact of medicine that will never change. That's the Last Commandment. All patients must be allowed to die."